Praise for *The Pain Companion*

"*The Pain Companion* is a practical, insightful, and compassionate guide for chronic pain sufferers. It is beautifully written and sensitive. For those who have searched to make sense of chronic pain, here is a packet of understanding — a place where hope and possibilities live."

— **Amber Wolf, PhD**

"I would call this the go-to book when nothing else works when you have chronic pain. The intuition, wisdom, exercises, and meditations offered by Sarah Anne Shockley are helpful beyond measure and can assist you on your journey to find your true self. This is a must-read book."

— **Michael A. DeFino, DC**

"*The Pain Companion* offers important insights into the world of chronic pain. Sarah Anne Shockley gives a comprehensive and profound look at the meaning within the experience of pain. I highly recommend this book for anyone, especially for people living with pain, caregivers, and medical and rehabilitation professionals."

— **Thaïs Mazur, OTR, PhD,** coauthor of *Do No Harm*

"*The Pain Companion* is a must-have for both pain sufferers and therapeutic practitioners practicing pain relief. Taking from her own life experience, Sarah Anne Shockley offers practical, deep, insightful ways of living with constant, twenty-four-hours-a-day pain, allowing readers ways to shift their mental, emotional, and physical approaches to pain management. I recommend *The Pain Companion* to all my chronic pain clients."

— **Dr. Celestine Star, DD, AH CH, BCI LC**

"A wise, thoughtful, heartfelt autobiography and manual. It beautifully lays out the negative emotions and limiting habits that so often accompany pain and offers strategies for coping and healing."

— **Carol Banquer, MD**

"It is so valuable to hear directly from someone who has lived through it herself and developed an approach to pain management that addresses all aspects of living in pain. I highly recommend this book for anyone living with pain or working with people in pain."

— **Pam Dent, OTR**

"*The Pain Companion* is an excellent resource and companion for those with pain. Learning how to become empowered through one's pain journey is incredibly important. Sarah Anne Shockley shares valuable insights and approaches to living with and managing chronic pain. This is a fantastic read."

— **Nicole Hemmenway,** vice president, U.S. Pain Foundation

"This very important book on making life with pain easier offers valuable advice and ideas that could only come from someone who has lived through it. I wholeheartedly recommend it to anyone experiencing chronic pain and suggest that practitioners read it to gain a greater understanding of the challenges their patients in pain live with."

— **Tracy A. Newkirk, MD**

The Pain Companion

The Pain Companion

Everyday Wisdom for Living With and Moving Beyond Chronic Pain

Sarah Anne Shockley

Foreword by Dr. Bernie S. Siegel

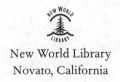

New World Library
Novato, California

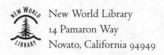

New World Library
14 Pamaron Way
Novato, California 94949

Text design by Tona Pearce Myers

Library of Congress Cataloging-in-Publication Data
Names: Shockley, Sarah (Sarah Anne) author.
Title: The pain companion : everyday wisdom for living with and moving beyond
    chronic pain / Sarah Anne Shockley.
Description: Novato, California : New World Library, [2018]
Identifiers: LCCN 2017061046 (print) | LCCN 2018001362 (ebook) |
    ISBN 9781608685714 (ebook) | ISBN 9781608685707 (alk. paper) |
    ISBN 9781608685714 (Ebook)
Subjects: LCSH: Pain—Alternative treatment. | Pain—Treatment.
Classification: LCC RB127 (ebook) | LCC RB127 .S487 2018 (print) |
    DDC 616/.0472—dc23
LC record available at https://lccn.loc.gov/2017061046

First New World Library printing, June 2018
ISBN 978-1-60868-570-7
Ebook ISBN 978-1-60868-571-4

Printed in Canada on 100% postconsumer-waste recycled paper

New World Library is proud to be a Gold Certified Environmentally Responsible Publisher. Publisher certification awarded by Green Press Initiative. www.greenpressinitiative.org

10   9   8   7   6   5   4   3   2   1

This book is dedicated to all those who have chosen
to release pain in themselves and in the world.

Contents

Part 3: Meditative Approaches to Physical Pain

Part 4: When Pain Is the Teacher

Foreword: Pain, the Unwanted Gift

Sarah Anne Shockley learned about pain the hard way, by experiencing it and being incapacitated by it. But she met the pain, and she worked with the pain, and she is offering you the benefit of her experience in this helpful, gentle book. Throughout the decades I have spent working with patients in all sorts of circumstances, I have described pain as an unwanted, but sometimes necessary, gift. At workshops I have often asked people if they would like to be free of all pain, both emotional and physical. When many have said yes, I have suggested that they may want to contact me in a few months or think about it a bit more. Those who sign up for what they think will be a gift — absence of all pain — may want to reconsider and cancel the supposed gift after they experience the problems associated with feeling no pain. For example, lepers and diabetics with peripheral neuropathy all too often lose their limbs because they cannot feel infections or injuries.

Also, think about our feelings and emotions and how important it is to respond to them. I grew up with a mother whose advice about every problem was always the same: "Do what will make you happy." She taught me to deal with my feelings, so today I have happy depressions. When I am hungry I seek nourishment, and when I feel gnawing unrest or other painful emotions I seek the changes in my life that will resolve the unhealthy and painful feelings. Experiencing and living with pain is one path in the journey of being a human, and *The Pain Companion* can help guide you along that journey.

Being open to experience what a journey offers is part of life. In support groups, I guide patients to draw what they are experiencing. I have found that when two people draw the same treatment, one might show it as hell and the other as heaven. If one patient depicts surgery as a mutilation and the operating room as a black box with a patient in it but no one caring for them, while another patient draws a life-saving gift from God showing flowers and the surgeon caring for the patient, the two patients' postoperative recovery will demonstrate the difference. I have done major surgery on people who have awakened and said, "I have no pain. I am a little sore." I explained to the nurses to please stop writing "Patient refuses pain medication" in their chart and instead write that the patient had no pain. Yet pain is present in many lives, and refuses to go away, and we must find ways to move through our lives despite the pain.

Studies reveal that when you put your hand in a bucket of ice and keep it there as long as possible, you can keep it in the ice longer if loved ones are standing by your side than if you are alone. And I bet you'd probably be able to keep it there even longer if your dog were present. I also know from personal experience with a back injury that when I was performing operations or painting a portrait — two activities where I lost track of time and was being loving and creative — I was not aware of my pain. When I stopped either activity, I needed to lie down because of the pain that I was now aware of once again. I think doing any activity that makes you lose track of time is the healthiest state you can ever be in.

I do not blame patients or deny that many painful syndromes require medications and various anesthetic therapies, but I am saying that one cannot separate the sensation from the individual and their life and beliefs. Two people with the same affliction do not necessarily experience and suffer the same degree of pain.

When we see life as a labor pain of self-birthing, the pain becomes meaningful and we no longer see it as a curse. For some it even becomes a blessing because of how it redirects their life toward finding nourishment for their body and soul. But when we are experiencing pain because of a prescribed treatment or a family member telling us that we must go through it to not die, we are in big trouble. We need to keep our power and find meaning in what we choose to do. I find that support groups are very helpful because the "natives" are able to share with one another and not be told what to do by the "tourists."

I experience pain, but I do not suffer. To me pain is a

necessity, but suffering is an option. When our pain has no meaning and does not lead to the healing of our life, we suffer greatly. But when we use our pain to become a more complete human being, the curse turns into a blessing. Let me close with a poem I received from a patient and teacher many years ago:

Nine months seems like a long time
I watch my body change
Tired I sit staring out at life
I live within my mind
Books and music transport me beyond my body
Nine months finally pass
I give birth to my child
All the discomfort and pain are now justified

Chemotherapy and radiation
Twelve months seems like a long time
I watch my body change
Tired I sit staring out at life
I live within my mind
Books and music transport me beyond my body
Twelve months finally pass
I give birth to myself
All the discomfort and pain are now justified

— Dr. Bernie S. Siegel, author of
The Art of Healing and *Love, Medicine & Miracles*

Introduction

I have lived with continuous, often intense physical pain since the fall of 2007. Every aspect of my life has been deeply affected, as certainly are the lives of those of you reading these words who also suffer from chronic pain.

Living in constant pain has been one of the most challenging things I have ever had to undergo in my life. It has been difficult, not only because of the physical suffering, but due to the intense emotional repercussions that accompany it. These emotional states include loss, grief, shame, and terror, and they can be nearly as demanding as the physical pain.

During this time, I have often felt isolated and alone. I did not have access to a support group, nor, if I had, did I feel well enough to attend one. You may find yourself in a similar situation. I have written this book to offer you the companion I wish I'd had, a guide on your journey to living with more ease and grace even in the midst of pain and, ultimately, to relieving and releasing pain.

The Pain Companion is not meant to replace conventional

physical remedies, medications, and procedures or the many excellent alternative healing modalities available today.

Instead, this book addresses the inner life of physical pain, how our responses to pain affect both its potency and longevity, and how that relationship has the potential to either contribute to prolonged suffering or provide a pathway to restoring health and well-being. It provides practical advice for living with chronic pain *and* for relieving suffering on mental, emotional, and physical levels.

How This Book Is Set Up

Part 1, "Pain Moves In," addresses the ways physical suffering affects our lives. It shines light on how pain moves in and takes over our experience and on how we respond to it.

Part 2, "The Emotional Life of Chronic Pain," addresses the very deep and persistent fears, anxieties, sadness, anger, and shame that living with chronic physical pain tends to engender, intensify, and hold in place.

These are the unseen but potent sides of pain that are seldom talked about and usually given very little room for expression. They include emotional, psychological, and spiritual dimensions that are very much interwoven with one another and with the nature of physical pain itself.

Part 2 also offers simple, practical steps to work with to help ease these psychological and emotional consequences of living with pain.

Part 3, "Meditative Approaches to Physical Pain," presents eleven meditative exercises I developed for myself to help open a path to physical relief and release. These are the most effective methods I have found to create a more beneficial and healing relationship with the pain in my body. More than any other approach offered by medical or therapeutic models, they helped reduce the amount of physical pain I was experiencing.

In part 4, "When Pain Is the Teacher," I present some of the most important life lessons I have learned with pain as my mentor, which offer invaluable insights for living life with more ease, grace, and wisdom. This section also discusses creating true healing and transformation in life while moving on from the place of pain.

I cannot know your personal suffering, of course; only you can. But I do understand the experience of being in significant and relentless pain for long periods of time, and I understand the fear, sadness, and frustration associated with long-term physical debilitation. So I can say that this book has been written from *inside* of pain, a perspective on the experience and the healing of pain that we are seldom offered.

I honor you for the courageous journey you are on. May these ideas help you cultivate deep compassion for yourself and aid you in finding increased well-being, peace, and solace as well as bodily relief.

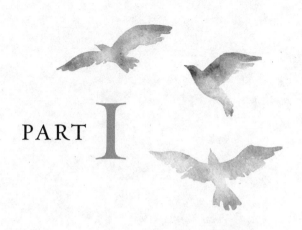

PART I

Pain Moves In

I   Life Taken Over by Pain

In the fall of 2007, I developed thoracic outlet syndrome (TOS) due to prolonged computer use in a nonergonomic office setup. Simply put, the area between my collarbones and first ribs collapsed, severely compressing the space to less than 20 percent of its normal width on both sides of my body.

This compression was excruciating, squeezing a major artery, veins, nerve ganglia, and the large scalene muscles running down from the neck to the first ribs, all of which must fit through this relatively small space.

This caused intense burning sensations in my neck; deep aches in my palms, wrists, and neck; and shooting pains in my neck and forearms. A continuous migraine headache often flared alarmingly, setting the right side of my brain on fire. I had flu-like dizziness, weakness, fatigue, and loss of mobility and functionality in my arms and hands.

Anything that required me to use my arms away from my body, even the smallest lifting, pushing, pulling, reaching, grasping, or carrying caused a sharp spike in pain levels. I could barely turn or tilt my neck to either side, up, or down, and I had to move my whole body slowly and carefully to look at someone next to me. I walked extremely slowly, leaning forward, like a very ancient person in bad shape.

In an effort to restore myself to health, I tried numerous approaches to healing, both traditional and alternative. Although some of them brought temporary relief, none actually healed the TOS, and the majority of them immediately made things worse by further irritating the nerves and tissues. After I tried a new approach, it usually took a number of days, and sometimes weeks, for the flare-up to calm down and the irritated nerves and swollen tissues to return to a more stable state.

Pharmaceuticals were also unsuccessful in relieving the nerve pain or aiding my overall condition. Instead, they created disagreeable side effects that added to the mélange of unpleasant symptoms already affecting most of my body, so I quickly stopped using them.

Since I couldn't dull the pain, I dulled myself instead and withdrew, becoming very still and quiet. It hurt to breathe deeply, so I sat propped up with pillows, my hands turned up and open, trying to breathe as lightly as possible and waiting for deliverance. If I waited long enough, I reasoned, the pain would go away and my body would receive the healing it needed through my careful stillness.

By the fall of 2008, I had been in intense, unceasing, and debilitating pain for the better part of a year, and I was not making any appreciable headway toward healing through either traditional or alternative methods. I felt as if I'd embarked on a nightmarish ocean liner heading out into dark and rough waters on a voyage with no predetermined destination and no way to disembark.

At first, I had thought everything was about to get better, and I would simply rejoin my life where I'd left off. It was an excursion I hadn't desired or asked for, but at least it would soon be over and I would carry on with life as usual. Every other malady I'd suffered had always ended. I had always healed before. Always.

But that's not what happened.

Many months passed before I fully understood the extent of my injuries. After an MRI scan and a series of diagnostics, my neurologist carefully explained that the extent of my TOS was unusually severe. Sadly, he informed me that I couldn't expect to heal anytime soon, if at all, and in fact, the condition was often progressive; it could steadily get worse.

In a two-hour consultation, a leading thoracic surgeon went over my status with me comprehensively, explaining that there really wasn't anything he could offer except a surgery of dubious merit in which my top two ribs would be removed. The recovery period would be very painful and protracted. And for me, it wouldn't be a permanent solution; I could expect my TOS to return.

These prognoses landed like dead weights. I had to come to terms with the fact that I would most probably not be returning to work or my normal activities. Ever. Along with living in pain, I realized that I was going to have to deal with the stress of making do with very reduced financial circumstances over a long period of time, as well as the ongoing sadness and distress of having had my normal, active life disappear, virtually overnight.

With the understanding that I was going to be physically impaired and in pain for a very long time, most likely the rest of my life, I entered a period of intense emotional challenge. My usual positive attitude faltered, and I began to experience decreased well-being and a constant barrage of worries about the future. I woke each day in the same dark state of mind, my body in extreme pain, and the condition of my life feeling the same, the same, the same, bleak morning after bleak morning.

Before my injury, I had considered myself resourceful, positive, intelligent, and capable. I certainly didn't expect others to figure things out for me. My inability to restore my body to health, therefore, was a source of deep frustration. Virtually everything I was doing to heal myself was leading nowhere constructive and often made things worse. What was I missing? What was I doing wrong?

✦

Dear Pain,

You have become such a forceful presence; it is almost like living with another person. My whole life has been hijacked by you. Other people say you come and go. You give them breaks for hours or days or even weeks, but you've decided to keep me company every single minute of every single day.

I realize now that the twinges and aches I felt at first were only your early scouts. Now you're here in full force — pressing, insistent, nasty, intense. You are unstoppable and all-pervasive. And you stay and stay and stay.

Why have you decided to stick with me so relentlessly, so adamantly, and with such passionate dedication?

※

2 The Submersion of the Self

When we experience severe pain, constant pain, insistent pain, the situation quickly becomes overwhelming. So much of our attention and energy is directed toward dealing with the pain that we can feel submerged underneath its demands.

The choices that have to be made, the responsibilities we still have despite a physical impairment, and the sensations of pain themselves seem to be drowning us. It becomes difficult to think clearly, to have conversations, to be available for life, to be available to the self.

Pain, therefore, rules our experience. It dictates how we can and can't use our bodies. We do only as much as it allows us to do. We sleep only as much as it allows us to sleep. When it has something to say, we are its captive audience. We interact with others with less enthusiasm and less energy. We become worn-out and discouraged, completely at the mercy of its whims.

Pain becomes our primary focus. That is its nature. Its

presence is all-encompassing. When pain is either very severe or very long-lived, it can feel like a separate entity, a being with its own mind.

It is like living with something or someone else in our bodies, a power unto itself, which we must serve. It has its own agenda and keeps its own schedules. Its needs are immediate and seemingly insatiable. We spend a great deal of time and energy bowing to it, taking care of it, trying to ease it, or imploring it to leave.

Tasks that were easy before become difficult and exhausting. Before the brain even attempts to tackle a problem or meet a demand, it feels overloaded and overwhelmed. Things that require a response — the phone, a question, paperwork — can seem like an invasion or attack. So little of us is left that is not overtaken by pain, there remains almost no energy with which to make decisions, to think, to feel, to love.

After living for days, weeks, and months with pain as the director of life, we can lose sight of our own primacy, and the primacy of other people and situations that are important or dear to us.

It's easy to feel irritable with everyone, with life, with ourselves. Part of the irritability is from the constant braying of nerves in pain, of course, but part is the frustration of not being able to control it. It feels like our bodies are no longer our own, and that is truly a very frightening invasion. It's too close, too intimate.

In addition, there are the stresses that accompany every waking moment, including the uncertainty about healing — if and when it will happen — and the unknowns of how to survive practically and financially.

We must face difficult questions, often meeting them with limited physical, mental, and financial resources: *What will happen if I can't take care of my children? What if I can no longer pay my mortgage or rent? Should I take a specific drug? Who will help me make sense of all these forms? How will I go shopping, do the laundry, clean? How can I afford to pay someone to help me?*

Being in constant physical pain is like living underwater. The pain sensations are not only felt in the body; they seem to become an extended energy field around the body, creating a separate reality that no one else shares.

There is no one inside your world of pain with you; you are utterly alone there. Even others who are also suffering do not share the same pain.

The sensation of pain, then, creates boundaries around the entire experience of life. It becomes the environment and the substance in which the self is immersed. The world recedes, often to a seemingly unreachable distance. Only echoes of it remain. Normal life seems remote; everything is filtered and distanced by the field of pain and the stress that comes with it, surrounding and penetrating all experience.

❧

Dear Pain,

I am trying everything I can think of to make you happy. To make you calm down. To make you go away. I have tried eradicating, releasing, relieving, mitigating, cajoling, begging, and ignoring you. Yet you are astonishingly resilient. You refuse to budge. Almost everything I do makes you louder and more insistent.

Today I was alarmed to discover that the only sensations I have left are painful ones. My entire body is a burning, painful structure. If there is a part of me that is not in pain, I can't feel it anymore. You have taken over my entire experience of my body!

Are you trying to push me out of my body? I don't believe I *am* this pain, but where am I? What is left of *me*?

❧

3   When Pain Won't Leave

Typically in Western medicine, one of the first things a doctor does for us when we're in physical pain is to provide medication or therapeutic treatment that eases the discomfort. A treatment is considered most successful if it not only addresses the physical ailment but substantially reduces or eradicates pain. In fact, in some cases, the only "cure" available to us is pharmaceutical pain relief.

Of course, most of us are very happy to be on the receiving end of pain relief when we need it. Having the goal of easing pain serves the important purpose of helping us become more comfortable so our bodies can rest and thereby heal more quickly. This is all well and good if the pain does end, the purpose is served, and we heal. However, as we well know, not all pain responds to medication and treatment.

When our doctors have run out of options and we continue to experience ongoing, even debilitating pain, when the level and duration of the pain tests the limits of our patience and our doctors' expertise, what then?

Because we generally treat all pain in the same way, and because we have the understandable, but unattainable, goal of ending all pain as quickly as possible, the persistence of pain can't help but imply a level of defeat.

When well-meaning doctors and therapists offer time-tables and expectations for our recovery that don't work out, it can oddly and unjustifiably feel like we are ailing in other ways: We aren't a good-enough patient, our bodies haven't responded correctly, something else is wrong with us, we're not normal, we must be malingering.

Our condition of continued pain can seem to morph from something unavoidable as a result of injury or illness into something unresolved and lingering, perhaps even appearing suspicious to others not experiencing it themselves.

This puts us in a very uncomfortable position. Because pain medications and healing protocols work on some kinds of pain, but not ours, we may feel that our chronic condition is a negative reflection on us: There is something wrong with us for continuing to experience pain.

We may feel abandoned by the medical establishment, which may metaphorically throw up its hands. Left to our own devices, we become, in many ways, our own last resort, yet we have no idea how to access the switch to turn the pain off.

Our distressing lack of clear movement toward healing is only underscored by the positive suggestions of others (*Have you tried X?*), the barrage of drugs we have taken to no avail, and the various treatments we have undergone with mixed or little success. It can appear that it isn't the drugs or the treatments that have failed, it's *us*.

When pain remains despite pharmaceuticals, physical therapies, surgeries, or other forms of therapeutic treatments and alternative modalities, instead of applying more of the same, we need to consider changing course altogether.

In my experience, short-term pain and chronic pain require very different approaches to relief and ongoing management. Chronic pain is a very complex condition involving much more than just the physical symptoms of the body. It includes emotional and psychological aspects as well, due to the incredible stresses of living with pain on a daily basis, and the ramifications of basically losing one's life to pain.

⚜

Dear Pain,

Why are you still here? I am frustrated and annoyed. I seem only to be getting worse, and you are not leaving. You, Pain, have moved in.

I didn't recognize the You of you for a full ten months. I treated you with respect, yes, but with the respect due a temporary lodger. I kept expecting you to leave. I dealt patiently with the extreme discomfort of your constant boarding because I assumed it was to be short-lived.

You are like a guest who shows up, unpacks in

the living room, pulls out an old brass horn, and starts playing loudly and out of tune. Tirelessly you play on day and night as if to discover who will wear out first. I have. I'm worn-out. Stop. Please. Just go away.

4 Feeling Bad about Feeling Bad

If your pain is new, you may still be in a degree of emotional and physical shock — shock from the illness or injury and shock from the trauma of having your affairs, your work, your life, and your relationships superseded by pain.

You may also suffer from post-traumatic stress disorder (PTSD). PTSD is a condition that occurs after severe stress, change, sudden loss, or injury — or, as I have found, from long-term disability, chronic pain, or a life-changing illness.

PTSD can cause you to become easily overwhelmed, highly irritable, disoriented, and terrified for no apparent reason and to suffer from insomnia and nightmares.

Living in pain for an extended period of time elicits its own strong emotional and psychological responses as well. These occur because of the physical discomfort we are in, obviously, but also because we are apparently losing the battle.

We are at the mercy of something that has moved in and taken over our experience. We fear that, in some hidden and insidious way, we are to blame for both its existence and our lack of success in making it all better.

Some of these intense emotional responses include grief, sadness, loss, shame, blame, resentment, failure, isolation, loneliness, and powerlessness. Because these emotions are powerful, and because they may live with us for as long as pain abides, they can eventually override our experience of ourselves and our lives.

They are understandable reactions to a life that has been overtaken by pain, but as time passes, we may lose our sense of who we really are.

Days of joy and ease recede into the distance, and it begins to seem as if we have always felt this bad. We have trouble remembering how to laugh freely, what our bodies felt like without pain, and what it was like just to feel generally okay.

Living with constant pain, I initially wanted to minimize any and all further suffering, so I tended to ignore or deny the emotional pain that I was also undergoing.

Ultimately, this was not a helpful choice. Over time, the experience of physical pain and our emotional responses to it can become interlocked, each cementing the other in place. They weave together like a Celtic knot, seemingly inextricable.

Some emotions are contractive reactions to pain. When we are locked in these emotional states, the body responds by tightening and contracting. This contraction of the body serves to further lock bodily pain in place.

It inhibits the free flow of breath and the free movement of life force and renewing energy through the body, and it impedes healing. Examples of feelings that tend to contract and tighten the body are resentment, bitterness, blame, and anger.

Emotions that drag us down and sap energy also inhibit the body's ability to heal. These emotions are like inner weights. They pull inward and downward, and we can feel as if we're living at the bottom of a well with no escape. These include hopelessness, self-pity, loss, and sadness.

In addition, we experience situational responses to pain that develop and establish themselves over time. I think of these as *feeling states*. They have emotional components but are experienced more as states of being. These include victimization, powerlessness, isolation, silence, and invisibility.

As a last-ditch effort born of the desperation of having no effective avenues of physical healing, I began working with these emotional aspects of living in pain. If I couldn't heal my body right away, I could at least work with the other levels of pain I was experiencing.

This began with the simple but surprisingly difficult practice of acknowledging the deep emotional pain that stemmed from, accompanied, and amplified my physical pain. From this place, I learned to extend compassion to myself.

This practice of extending understanding and compassion to myself was more than just a psychological wellness exercise. It was a crucial interior movement that created space for real healing and unexpectedly began to relieve my physical pain as well.

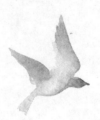

PART 2

The Emotional Life
of Chronic Pain

5 Pain's Emotional Traps

Part 2 explores the ways that physical pain takes over our emotional experience, how it affects our quality of life, and our relationships with ourselves and others. It addresses the difficult emotions that accompany living in physical pain and provides suggestions to help relieve them, thereby beginning to unravel the knot of suffering.

Lessening the sense of loss, sadness, guilt, and shame engendered by chronic pain serves to create more emotional space and fosters the resilience needed for living with physical pain and, ultimately, for easing that pain.

Each section in part 2 discusses a particular emotion or feeling state and then offers "antidotes" for how you might work through them. These antidotes are suggestions only, not a prescription. They are coping strategies that I found worked for me. I have used them continually over the course of ten years, some all the time and some for only brief periods.

However, not all of them will be applicable to your

situation. You may not use all of them, of course, or even any of them, if you find they don't suit your needs. Modify them as you wish. Some may inspire you to think of your own.

As you read the following pages, strong feelings may come up in response to the material presented. This may be the first time you have allowed yourself to feel the emotional side of physical pain.

Deep feelings that are not allowed to be acknowledged, I have found, do not simply leave on their own and may be locking physical pain in place.

Take it slow, be kind to yourself, and know that feeling your emotions does not mean you are creating them. If you are feeling them now, they are already present, and it is best to give them a little space to be experienced, rather than to ignore them, so they can complete themselves and move on.

The "Technique for Releasing Difficult Emotions," which follows, can be used anytime strong, difficult, or unexpected emotions arise.

TECHNIQUE FOR
RELEASING DIFFICULT EMOTIONS

Step 1. Notice Your Emotion or Feeling State
Step 2. Feel
Step 3. Breathe from Inside the Emotion
Step 4. Notice the Spaciousness
Step 5. Decide if You're Ready to Feel Differently
Step 6. Notice the Change

Step 1. Notice Your Emotion or Feeling State

Notice the specific emotion or feeling state that accompanies your physical pain as it arises. This could include sadness, grief, anger, helplessness, self-pity, numbness, or a host of other responses. Just allow both the emotional response and the physical pain to be there together for now, and notice how they exist side by side or perhaps intertwined.

Step 2. Feel

Step inside your emotional state, allowing yourself to feel it as fully as you can for a few moments. As you allow yourself to feel your emotions fully, is your physical pain heightened? Diminished? Unaffected?

Step 3. Breathe from Inside the Emotion

Let yourself breathe into and through your feelings, continuing to notice your physical pain at the same time. From *inside the emotion*, breathe in and through, in and through your experience.

Step 4. Notice the Spaciousness

Still breathing in and through the emotional state, begin to notice a growing spaciousness. There is still the intensity of the feeling, but there is also the spaciousness of the breath. The spaciousness is there with the emotion, around the emotion, and infusing the emotion with breath. Include all of that in your experience.

Step 5. Decide If You're Ready to Feel Differently

Decide if you are ready to feel differently about your pain, your situation, and yourself right now. Don't try to resolve anything or answer all your questions about why or how it all happened or is happening; just decide whether or not you are ready for a change. Take a deep breath, if you can, and release it fully. Let the emotion release, subside, or expend itself for now.

Step 6. Notice the Change

Notice how this cycle affects both your emotional and physical pain levels as you work with it repeatedly.

6   Guilt and Shame

It doesn't make logical sense that we would feel guilty about being ill or injured and in pain, yet we often do.

Our modern culture puts a premium on keeping up, carrying on, being strong, not complaining, and toeing the line. We leave almost no room for the body's need for rest and true refreshment and relaxation. Even our vacation time is short and filled with activity.

We do not have a philosophy of regular downtime dedicated to physical regeneration or of the natural daily cycles of rest and quiet that support true wellness. In fact, it is almost a sin to do nothing, to step out of the constant stream of work, entertainment, and busyness.

We worry that if we allow ourselves to withdraw from activity and participation in the game of life for more than a very brief interlude, we are simply not good people. Good people take short breaks and then keep going and keep trying; they never give up and never say die.

When we are forced to stop and rest due to a physical infirmity, therefore, we often feel bad about it. We think we should be up and around; we should be on the phone with people at work; we should be taking care of things. If we are still working or responsible for family, we may feel we must hide our pain, pretend it isn't there, and do as much as we would normally do. We think we must "grin and bear it."

Since we do not have a positive context for pain as a natural element of the process of healing and recovery, we see it only as something to fight, overcome, and eventually eradicate. If we can't do that, we're somehow letting ourselves be run by the enemy. We feel guilty when we can't make it stop, when we can't quickly return to our lives, our duties, and our commitments.

We are under pressure to heal for all kinds of reasons: We want to get back to work, our kids need our attention, our relationships are strained, the medical bills are piling up, we're tired of being in pain, and so on.

Doctors, therapists, workers' compensation systems, and insurance companies often have an expectation for what they feel is an appropriate amount of time within which our bodies are expected to heal. If we aren't responding positively to treatments, or we simply require a more lengthy recovery period than is considered the norm, we not only feel pressure to heal faster but we can feel shame for not having healed already.

Not healing, not releasing our bodily ills and pain, creates guilt because in some way we feel like it's our fault that things aren't working out better. We worry that we're not doing enough to heal, that we aren't trying hard enough.

We may feel on some deep level that we are letting ourselves and everyone else down. We are concerned that we are burdening others as well. We don't want our loved ones to worry, and we want to relieve them of having to do the things we can't do for ourselves.

As the amount of time we are in pain and unable to work lengthens, we may experience a subtle, creeping, persistent feeling of shame and failure.

Eventually, we may feel like we are somehow less than a whole person, since we are unable to fully contribute to and participate in life. This can lead to feelings of depression, uselessness, and meaninglessness.

Antidotes to Guilt and Shame

Recognize That You Are Not Wrong for Being in Pain

One of the first things to understand is that being in pain is not your fault. You are not wrong, guilty, bad, or screwed up.

The fact that you can't turn pain off doesn't mean that you aren't trying hard enough or that, in some unconscious way, you *want* to continue to suffer. Accidents happen, illness happens, pain happens. They are part of living life on Earth as a human being. No one lives their entire life without facing some of these challenges.

So the first step in relieving guilt and shame is to allow yourself to know that being in pain does not equate with being weak, bad, or needy, nor does it mean you are wrong or inadequate as a person.

Remember That You Are Not on Anyone's Timetable

As much as we want to be promised a time frame within which our pain will cease, and we want to be able to promise others that we will be fully recovered by a certain date, the truth is that our bodies are on their own healing schedule, which can't be forced.

Pain keeps its own timetables, and no one has the ability to read them completely accurately, not even your doctor. Right now, take a deep breath and then release it fully, letting go of the need to heal by a certain date.

Pain will stay as long as it needs to, and your job is to learn to listen and respond to your physical and emotional needs. Let go of the pressure you are putting on yourself to end the pain right now this minute.

You simply can't force healing. It is not productive and leads to resentment toward others who are trying to help, toward your own body, and toward yourself.

Be a little kinder to yourself, relax more, and allow yourself to be right where you are right now. Then decide to give your body the time it needs to truly heal.

Drop the Guilt about Needing Help

While in pain, your ability to handle the everyday tasks of life is automatically compromised. It's part of the package.

First, recognize that if you're in pain, you need help. The kind of help you need may be physical, such as shopping or rides to the doctor, but you may also need emotional support in the form of a shoulder to cry on or someone who will just listen to you vent for a while.

Everyone has times in life when they need to depend on others for help in various forms and to varying degrees. This is your time.

Be as grateful and gracious about it as you can be, but drop the guilt about receiving support. It turns out that most people are happy to help. In fact, they feel better about themselves after they have helped someone else.

I had to learn not only to ask for help from friends and family but that it was okay to ask strangers to open doors, pull out chairs, carry groceries, or reach for something out of range.

If it's really hard for you not to feel guilty about asking for help from others, make a pact with yourself that, once you are well enough, you will repay others directly in some form, or that you will find at least one other person in need and contribute to their well-being in whatever way you can.

Make Lists of People You Can Call On

When we're in pain, everything is more difficult. Do yourself a favor and, when you've got a little bit of energy, make a list of friends, family, and professionals and their contact information.

This list will include people who can potentially help you when you need it. Subdivide your main list into three shorter lists (A, B, and C), according to people's availability.

A-list people are those you feel you can rely on to do

their best to be available for you as often as possible. It includes best friends, close family, and any others who are able and willing to do physical tasks as well as to provide solace and companionship.

B-list people are friends, family, neighbors, and members of organizations that you belong to who have offered to help or who seem like people who could help out occasionally.

C-list people are backup people to call on rarely or only in a pinch when you can't reach anyone else. These might include those who are usually too busy with kids and career to be helpful but who might be able and willing to make an effort in an emergency.

When you're in deep pain, down in the dumps about your situation, or both, these lists can be an incredible life raft. Just knowing you have them is an emotional boost.

Also, having others to call outside of your normal helpers and caregivers (often family) can give those people a break they may well need. There may also be nonprofit organizations in your area that can meet some of your needs at little or no cost.

Ask for Help Clearly and Honestly

Ask for the help you need as clearly and honestly as you can. Sometimes shame and guilt about needing help makes us reluctant to ask, so we mask it. Either we don't ask or we ask in such a roundabout way that it feels manipulative and can be annoying to others.

For example, if you need a ride to the doctor, don't call a friend and casually mention that you have an appointment next Tuesday and you're not sure how you'll get there, hoping they will offer. It's much better to be up-front and clear about what you need. Simply ask if they are available and willing to give you a ride and give them an accurate estimate of how long it will take. This gives others an opportunity to say yes or no, and it shows respect for them and their time.

Most of us remain vague about our needs because we are afraid that people will say no, and we don't want to be disappointed. We don't want to find out that others aren't really there for us.

When you're in pain and in need of support, however, it's important to get over these fears. You'll find out who is available and who isn't. Don't blame those who are unable or unwilling to help, and do be appreciative of those who are.

Receive Financial Assistance Graciously

Some of us feel guilty about receiving financial assistance when we need it, whether from family, government, or other agencies.

One pervasive perception we have in our culture is that people who accept assistance are mooching off society. This can make it uncomfortable when you find yourself in a situation in which you must rely on outside financial help. It is, however, part of the natural give-and-take of life.

Sometimes we put money in the collective pot, and

sometimes we need to draw money out. If you're receiving government assistance, you've been paying into the system for the duration of your work life, and it is *supposed* to be there for you when you need it.

If it's charity, then the money has come from people like you who willingly give to help others. If it's from family, accept what is given, graciously and with gratitude, and do your best to repay it, if and when you are able.

Stop Making Other People Feel Better

Let go of needing to make other people feel emotionally better because they can't make you feel physically better.

This advice is for your immediate family and friends, but it also extends to your doctors and therapists. They may have a desire for you to get better that puts unintended pressure on you to heal more quickly.

While it's only natural that others want you to heal, it is not your responsibility to take care of them emotionally.

Making other people feel better can take the form of (a) not expressing what you need so you don't burden them, (b) downplaying your continued pain so your doctor or other caretakers feel better about the job they're doing, or (c) attempting programs or exercises that you're not ready for because you are responding to someone else's urging or avoiding blame for not trying harder.

The best remedy is to remain clear and honest. As appropriate, tell people:

This doesn't work for me.

I am not feeling any improvement.

I am not ready for that yet.

Please respect that I am doing everything I can to heal, and it will take the time it takes.

The best thing you can do for me now is trust my healing process.

Know That Healing Is Your Current Job

Being in pain from illness or injury, you may not be able to work to your full capacity, if at all, but this doesn't mean that what you're doing at this time is not important.

What's true is that your current career has shifted for the moment. Your real job, for now, is healing.

Don't judge yourself harshly according to what you used to be capable of doing. You are handling another aspect of life right now that requires a great deal of time and energy.

Make feeling better a higher priority than keeping up with your previous goals. Those will have to be on hold for now. Take advantage of sick leave and whatever assistance you require to make a full recovery, and never feel guilty about your needs.

When you heal, you will have a stronger sense of appreciation for the life you have and a greater capacity for compassion for yourself and others.

Your priorities may be rearranged for a while, or forever, but that's not always a bad thing. Let yourself learn whatever this time with pain is trying to teach you.

SUMMARY

- You are not wrong for being in pain.
- You are not on anyone's timetable.
- Drop the guilt about needing help.
- Make lists of people you can call on.
- Ask for help clearly and honestly.
- Receive financial assistance graciously.
- Stop making other people feel better.
- Know that healing is your current job.

7   Anger and Blame

While guilt and shame often stem from a belief in our own failings, anger and blame usually arise when we look outward and try to understand our situation from the standpoint of the people and circumstances that seem to have caused our problems.

When we're not getting better, when we're in pain and it is relentless, sooner or later we are going to get angry at someone or something.

We ask, *Why me? How did this happen? Who or what is to blame for my misery?* We look for the root so we can understand what happened. We think that if we can understand how it all came about, we can somehow undo it.

The trouble with this mindset is that the only way to answer these questions is to find something to blame: the job, the boss, the stresses of life, the other driver, the doctors who didn't see it coming, air pollution, fatty foods, genetics, a traumatic childhood, our spouse, or anything else we can think of. We imagine that there is one thing, one starting point, one cause. If we can find it, we can heal.

At times, it is useful to pinpoint the onset of pain, such as when knowing exactly how an injury or illness happened can contribute to returning to wellness. But once that is found, it is no longer helpful to continually go over the history of an injury or ailment, the mistakes, or who was responsible for what.

No matter the real cause of your situation, at some point, you are also going to feel angry with yourself for having gotten into this situation, for making the choices that somehow led to this.

You can also build up resentment against yourself for not being able to get out of the fix you are in. It just seems to reflect badly on you as a person.

Of course, most people will say that they don't think less of you because you are in pain or don't consider you a bad person for being sick or injured. But *you* may.

On the inside, you feel awful about having to live in this situation and inflicting it on others. You can't help it. It wears on you and can create a negative sense of self over time.

You will undoubtedly also feel angry at the pain because it is so insistent and so faceless, a force that can't be bribed, cajoled, or bargained or reasoned with.

Anger is understandable, and it can be very healthy, but keeping it around because you need someone or something to blame, including yourself, only serves to keep pain in place.

Antidotes to Anger and Blame

Allow Your Anger, Then Use It for Fuel

There is nothing inherently wrong with feeling angry about what happened and what you are currently suffering. In fact, for people stuck in depression and sadness, anger can be a very liberating force.

Anger has a lot of energy in it. Rather than sitting still and feeling powerless, anger wants to move and change things, so it can be a very helpful emotion when harnessed for good. It can move people out of the doldrums and into positive action.

However, once you have gotten in touch with anger, you don't want to stay in it. It's not helpful to continuously feel angry and blaming, even if there is something specific to fault. It simply isn't conducive to healing.

Anger that doesn't move turns to bitterness. Use its energy to fuel your determination to recover, rather than let it eat away at you. Let it go and you are free to move on.

Leave the Past Where It Is

If it is important to you, spend the time you need to make a clear assessment of how your illness or injury came to be, then leave it alone. If the cause is uncertain or a complete mystery, then make the choice to leave it as a mystery for the time being.

Your energy and attention need to be on healing, not

on who did or didn't do something, or what exact circumstances were at fault. With the only exception being the times you may need to be involved in legal activities or a medical review, or if the cure lies in finding the exact cause, leave the past in the past.

The energy of blame is always looking backward, and you need to marshal your resources in the present so you can heal and have a better future.

Let Go of Resentments

I think of resentment as the quieter cousin of blame. Rather than accusing and pointing the finger, resentment seems to stem from a creeping and pervasive sense of unfairness.

I noticed that I sometimes felt resentful that I was injured through my employment, but my employer was able to carry on with life as usual. I resented his freedom and normalcy, while I had to live with pain and debilitation day in and day out as a result of working for him. I felt it was somehow unfair that he carried on relatively unscathed (except for some financial ramifications).

I resented having a doctor I had never seen before spend about thirty minutes with me and write a report that strongly influenced my disability settlement. I resented the way the workers' compensation and disability system required me to keep re-proving my injury over and over again instead of actually supporting me to heal.

Keeping these feelings around wasn't going to get me anywhere positive. I had to learn to notice them when they arose and then decide to just let them go. In the interests of your own well-being, I would recommend letting go of resentments against anyone involved who has hindered your healing or given you bad advice or seems to be unsupportive. You just don't have the energy to waste on blame and resentment. Instead, use your energy for healing yourself.

Hold Everyone and Everything Blameless

As a second step to releasing resentments, decide to relieve everyone and everything of their burden of blame, including yourself, even if you feel blame is deserved.

This can be challenging because many of our legal and insurance systems can be very adversarial, bent on finding out who is to blame, and we speak of pain, illness, and injury as if they are enemies to be overcome. It is easy to fall into that pattern, but it really isn't a useful strategy for healing.

The point isn't whether or not you're *right* and justified, which may well be the case. The point is that holding on to anger, blame, and resentment simply isn't going to get you where you want to go.

SUMMARY

- Allow your anger, then use it for fuel.
- Leave the past where it is.
- Let go of resentments.
- Hold everyone and everything blameless.

8 Victimization and Powerlessness

One of the most challenging things for me about being injured and in pain was the powerlessness I felt because I was unable to heal my body and unable to stop the constant pain.

I also felt beholden to outside authorities: the medical system, the workers' compensation system, the legal system, and the disability system.

It's easy to feel you have lost control over your own destiny if you are required to rely on anything or anyone outside yourself to make a determination about your circumstances.

You may have family members and good friends who believe in you or a doctor or health practitioner who is especially understanding, yet none of them are powerful enough to make things go back to the way they were before. None of them can wave a magic wand and make everything work out with your finances and your medical coverage, and none of them can tell you what the perfect choices are that will ensure that you heal.

You may feel victimized by your condition, pharmaceuticals, invasive procedures, the impersonality of most institutions, or your own body. You may feel you are at the mercy of an interlocking system of agencies and organizations, none of which may present a caring or compassionate face.

Medical and insurance forms, appointments, tests, procedures, and legal hearings don't take into account that you are not at your best mentally and emotionally, that you are in terrible pain, or that you have very little stamina, yet you may feel blamed if you are not on top of the situation or able to answer questions clearly and accurately.

Sometimes, being ill or injured feels like it has become a crime committed by you.

Antidotes to Victimization and Powerlessness

Notice What You Can Control

In an effort to feel less at the mercy of outside forces and more in control of my life, I started noticing the decisions I had that were still under my control.

I noticed the decisions I was already making and congratulated myself for them. I also looked at the ones that I had handed over to others because I didn't know I could make them for myself, or I hadn't felt I had the knowledge or strength to make them, and I took them back.

In short, I recognized the self-empowerment I was already wielding and added to it.

Take Responsibility

Believing that others are responsible (or guilty) places them in a position of power and positions you as the victim.

To leave the world of powerlessness behind, I decided that, regardless of the circumstances of my injury, I was responsible for my situation from that point forward.

I declared myself at the center of my own emotional and physical well-being and recovery. I decided not to accept an outside source as the final authority, no matter how credible.

I knew that I was the one who would ultimately heal myself anyway, regardless of the method used. That decision alone, while not bringing with it an instantaneous and miraculous cure, at least afforded a measure of relief and a feeling of having more access to different choices rather than living entirely at the mercy of outside authorities and systems.

Choose Your Healing Path

With whatever energy you have, spend some time on the internet researching your condition (or ask someone to do it for you) so you can make informed decisions about treatment.

Look for alternative therapies, natural healing, recent research, and the latest medical breakthroughs. Read blogs and stories about how other people are coping with your condition and how some have cured themselves.

Decide for yourself how you will handle recommended

medications and procedures. Whatever advice you end up taking, notice that you are *choosing* that path for yourself; you are *choosing* that person's expertise and *choosing* whether to follow through.

Find out what you can do for yourself: how improving your diet can help healing, how you can think more positively, what herbs and supplements might be beneficial, how you can reduce the amount of stress you're under, and how you can get more restful sleep.

SUMMARY

- Notice what you can control.
- Take responsibility.
- Choose your healing path.

9   Fear, Anxiety, and Stress

When healthy, many of us take our bodies for granted most of the time. We're not surprised to wake up in the morning and be in a body that works generally well. We get up and go about our day not worrying if we can put one foot in front of the other. In fact, basic body functioning is usually the least of our worries. We're so sure of our bodies, we often pay minimal attention to them until they show signs of distress.

However, since the body is our vehicle for being in life and for participating in life, when we can't rely on it, it's incredibly frightening. All of a sudden everything changes.

When the body is not functioning properly, it brings up a huge amount of fear and anxiety. We can't wake up in the morning and assume everything is going to be all right. In fact, things may be very, very *not* all right.

Anxieties begin to multiply as the length of time in pain increases. You get the double whammy of needing to rest and relax so you can heal, but you don't feel relaxed at all because of ongoing work and family demands.

With prolonged time away from work comes the stress of not being able to keep up with what needs to be done. Tasks already put off for a week or two become critical, but you don't know how you will handle them with your body still compromised.

You may become worried about things falling apart without you, missing advancement opportunities, or the possibility that you may never go back to work at all.

Other stresses come from dealing with medical appointments, insurance companies, child-care arrangements, medical bills, and demands from family or partners. It seems hugely unfair that, at the time when you most need to rest and heal, your anxieties are mounting.

I often woke up in the middle of the night with panic attacks from survival terrors. I didn't know if I would be approved for ongoing disability funds, how I would live with a body that wasn't employable, or how I was going to meet even the simplest demands of life.

Being totally stressed-out and worried made the level of pain in my body skyrocket, so I had to find some way of working with the tension, anxiety, and fear.

Antidotes to Fear, Anxiety, and Stress

Acknowledge That Fear Is Not a Creative Force

Fear naturally arises when you are living in pain because so many unanswerable questions remain about the possibility of things getting even worse; how and if the pain will subside; and when, how, and if you will get better.

Fear is a natural reaction to the unknown, particularly if you are feeling less than fit physically, but all in all, I find it to be an unhelpful response. As I eventually realized, stressing out about my situation does not actually help it. For one thing, fear does not bring anything positive with it. It is not a creative force.

Fear does not change anything except to add more stress to the situation. No amount of worry is going to reorganize the world or fix anything. In fact, being anxious usually makes any physical condition worse.

Our minds worry over the future because we think that worrying is actually *doing* something. We think that if we're not worried, it means we don't care. But fear, worry, and anxiety do not actually produce positive results. They sap energy.

Employ the Fear Protocol

On the following page is my Fear Protocol. It's the method I created for myself to help reduce the terrors and anxiety of panic attacks. After you read through it and use it a couple of times, it's easy to remember the five steps. They will become second nature. Use them anytime you feel anxious or afraid, day or night. Allaying fear is a discipline of the mind, and I find this technique to be immensely helpful.

SUMMARY

- Fear is not a creative force.
- Employ the Fear Protocol.

THE FEAR PROTOCOL

Step 1. Notice What's Really Happening

Step 2. Notice What Has Already Worked Out

Step 3. Notice What You Can Take Charge Of

Step 4. Notice What's Going Well Right Now

Step 5. Time It and Start Again

Step 1. Notice What's Really Happening

Tell your mind that you are leaving your worry alone for a moment. Know that it will still be there if you want to go back to it later.

Fear is always about the future. It's about what might happen. Notice that what you're afraid of probably isn't happening in this moment and may never happen. In fact, most of the things we worry about never actually occur.

Step 2. Notice What Has Already Worked Out

Consciously calm your breathing and go back in time to the last thing you were really worried about. Notice how much of your worrying helped. Did worry have a direct positive impact on the outcome? Did it work out the way it worked out regardless of the amount of time you spent in fear and anxiety?

Also, notice that, one way or another, it did work out. Go back over the last several weeks and months and look at the things that caused you a great deal of anxiety and notice how many of them have already worked themselves out better than you feared. For now, you are still alive and carrying on. Go back to earlier in the day and notice if what you are worried about happened yet today.

Now, to whatever degree you can muster, allow yourself to trust that things will work themselves out this time, too, one way or another. Sometimes it will be in ways you want, sometimes not, and sometimes it will work out even better than you thought.

Step 3. Notice What You Can Take Charge Of

Since fear seems to come from feeling out of control of the situation, pay attention to what you can take charge of. You are ultimately in charge of how you feel, for one. It is your choice to be in fear and anxiety or to find a way to trust in life. Consider how you can be proactive and take charge of the decisions you need to make today and to-morrow. Make one firm decision right now, even if it is a relatively minor one.

Step 4. Notice What's Going Well Right Now

Consciously relax and breathe as calmly as you can. Find something to be grateful about that is happening right now in the moment and put your attention there. Find anything, even if it's the fact that your sheets are clean, or you can hear a nice breeze outside, or the neighbors have stopped shouting.

Notice the systems already in place that are working for you. In your mind's eye, see the people who are helpful to you and say thank you to them one by one: your doctor, your friends, your family, your coworkers.

If you are getting any financial assistance whatsoever, acknowledge that help to yourself and say thank you inside. If you've noticed any improvements in your condition, say thank you.

If the people you love are doing well, say thank you. If things could be worse than they are now, notice that they aren't and say thank you. Say thank you for all the things that could have gone wrong and didn't.

Step 5. Time It and Start Again

Go back to worrying if you really need to. Take exactly five minutes to worry excessively without making yourself wrong for it. Stop immediately when the time is up. Work through the protocol from the top again until you feel better. End on a positive note.

IO Isolation and Loneliness

Chronic pain can be very isolating. You may have very few people to talk to who understand what it is like to live in constant pain. There may be no welcoming place to speak openly about your fears and difficulties with those who are meeting similar challenges and who will not feel sorry for you or try to fix you.

Being in pain is like living in a different world. There is a sensitive bubble around you that others cannot fully recognize and understand. The painful sensations are felt in the body, but they also seem to inhabit the air around you, as if hypersensitive nerve endings extend a few feet from your body and make the space around you feel like it is part of your pain world.

When you are in severe pain, someone getting too close physically can set alarm bells off in your body before they have even touched you. This adds to the feeling of being cut off from others and the world by this painful enclosure and, in a way, *needing* to be cut off.

In addition, you may contract yourself physically in order to keep yourself safe from the haphazard movements of others that might poke or knock against you. You may also contract yourself emotionally, withdrawing from others by choice or necessity.

If you have restricted mobility, or your condition is debilitating in other ways, you can feel even more isolated. Being unable to participate meaningfully, you may feel very disconnected from the world, life, and others. You are still alive and *in* life, yet you don't feel nearly as much an active *part* of life. This sense of separation from others and from the world can feel extremely lonely.

When you are in pain, you are also more tired and groggy than usual. The added sensation of being "out of it" and in a fog makes it feel like you're always in a kind of jet-lagged state. Socializing can be challenging because putting out the energy to converse and act normally is often exhausting.

Whether your condition limits interactions because you are bedridden or less than fully mobile in other ways, or if you are mobile but in significant pain, you feel the limitations on your ability to truly be with others the way you usually enjoy. You talk less, leave early, withdraw more, or stop going out much at all, even if you can. In either case, pain becomes closer to you than any other companion, and your normal, carefree interactions with others can seem like only a memory.

Antidotes to Isolation and Loneliness

Don't Cut Yourself Off

You might feel that the best way to deal with the limitations imposed by deep pain is to simply stop socializing altogether, but over the long run, this may not be a healthy choice. You may certainly need to limit how much you go out if it exhausts you or increases your pain. You will need to become an expert at monitoring your own energy and pain levels so that you don't overdo it.

Obviously, some activities you will simply not be up for. At a dinner party, for example, let people know you'll only be able to stay for part of the evening or will arrive later for a bit of dessert.

Choose social events that will not wear you out. Be aware of how much energy you have and what increases your pain level and choose judiciously. Say no to events that are too crowded, too long, too loud, or in any way too demanding of you. Let friends and family know not to take it personally if you have to cancel or postpone at the last minute.

Here are some simple suggestions for being with others while taking care of your pain levels:

- Have a friend drive you wherever you're going and ask them to be flexible about how long you stay. If they know you well, they may help you monitor your energy level. Leave before you're exhausted, not after.

- Find social activities that don't tax your body, and let others wait on you. For example, plan a movie night at your home and ask your friends to organize the food and movie and to clean up after.

- Tone down the volume and visit quiet places. Choose to go with a friend who understands your limitations and is willing to leave as soon as you give the signal. Such places include bookstores, museums, art galleries, and quiet cafés.

- If you have the energy, start a group for people who suffer from chronic pain and arrange to meet for an hour at a local café to just talk and share a cup of tea or coffee. Or research online to see if there are any existing groups in your area.

- Look for talks or music events at your local library or coffeehouse that offer something interesting but won't tax you as much as a large, noisy venue.

In short, instead of staying home because you can't do the things you used to do, modify your outings to suit your physical needs and invite an understanding friend or two to join you.

Organize Regular Visits

If you can't get out, or if going out is too exhausting, phone or email friends to come by and visit, or ask a family member to contact a list of close friends for you. Choose times when you are apt to be most energetic and organize regular short visits from friends.

Your friends will usually feel good about having a clear way to help and to keep a connection with you. Let them know what you are capable of in terms of length of time and any activities you can participate in, or if you just want to chat. Ideas for simple activities with friends might include reading aloud installments of a novel by your favorite author, working on a jigsaw puzzle or crossword together, playing cards, discussing events at work or in the neighborhood, sharing a home-cooked meal, watching a movie, posting updates on social media, or listening to music. If your friends ask if there is anything they can do to help while they're there, say yes! Have a list of small tasks they can choose from.

These tasks could include quick cleaning (wiping kitchen counters, dusting or vacuuming a room); making a light meal; doing some shopping or laundry; picking up prescriptions; helping you read and fill out forms; answering emails or making phone calls for you; or doing research on your condition on the internet. More energetic friends can scrub your bathtub, mop floors, or cook full meals to freeze for later use.

Try Alternative Avenues for Socializing

There are also other ways of interacting with friends and continuing to feel part of life if you aren't up for long conversations or you can't know when you'll feel well enough for a visit.

If you are able to use a computer, use social media — such as Facebook, Twitter, Instagram, or Pinterest — to help you feel a little more connected. You can see what others are up to and pick and choose any interactions, keeping them brief.

Talking with friends on Skype, Zoom, or Google Hangouts is also a good way to connect; it feels more intimate than just speaking on the phone, since you can see each other. There are also numerous other ways to interact online, such as joining a chat group or blog discussing your favorite topic, joining an online group of people who are dealing with the same or a similar condition, or taking an easy online course that includes interactive chats with other students.

Use Nature's Solace

Spending time outside in trees or by water really helps restore a sense of connection with all of life. I try to spend a minimum of thirty minutes outside every day, either walking or sitting near trees.

I listen to the breeze, to the birds, to the creaking woods, to the rustle of small animals, to my breath. I find it very calming, and it reminds me that I am still alive and that life is still all around me in all its forms, no matter how my body feels. When I can, I arrange to meet a friend who doesn't mind walking slowly and for a limited distance.

Practice Positive Presence

Being in pain, I didn't feel as friendly as usual and frowned more often. It felt like pain had created its own atmosphere around me, and it was acting as a shield toward the world.

When I did interact with others, it was always through the pain and seemingly from a distance created by that pain.

But I decided that, even though I couldn't stop the physical discomfort I was in, I didn't have to withdraw from others completely. I could be present in my life despite the pain. I began to initiate small conversations with other people in line at the coffee shop or grocery store, with checkout people and neighbors. The conversations were necessarily brief, but I made a practice of making them as sincere as I could. I found it made me feel better to smile more, and it made people around me feel better, too.

When I am with my son, instead of noticing how much pain I am in, what I can't do, and how tired I am, I try to focus on him. I focus on being very present with him. I laugh more. I try to be very *there* when I interact with others, and in that way I am more available to people around me, if only briefly.

Through this practice, I've noticed that I can still have a positive effect on others, even when I feel like hell. It's a challenge because of the pain and because of the sense of distance pain creates, as if you are talking through a fog, but it helps. These things can shift my feelings of loneliness and isolation. I have found that I don't have to be healed or pain-free to find ways to remain part of the life going on around me.

SUMMARY

- Don't cut yourself off.
- Organize regular visits.
- Try alternative avenues for socializing.
- Use nature's solace.
- Practice positive presence.

I I Invisibility and Silence

Some injuries and illnesses are obvious, visible, and easily recognizable. Pain, however, remains unseen except as it affects the way someone holds their body, their demeanor, or their outward expressions.

As with love, hatred, caring, or jealousy, we might see evidence of its presence, but we cannot see the feeling itself. Those on the outside cannot weigh it or measure it or truly prove or disprove its presence. Pain, its level and sensation, is a uniquely private experience.

Because our pain is so much a part of what shapes our current experience, and because it is invisible to others, a feeling of invisibility can migrate over to our sense of self and *we* can begin to feel unseen as well.

Furthermore, many of us do not want to burden others, nor do we want them to feel like they can't keep us company without hearing an endless litany of complaints or a catalogue of our symptoms. For anyone who is in pain and who is considerate of the time, feelings, and concern of others, an awareness of how much we are asking of family, friends, and caretakers is always present. So we respond to inquiries in as positive a way as possible and turn the conversation away from our situation.

This is not a bad thing in itself; it certainly can be wearying to others to hear our plight repeated over and over. Yet consistently keeping this silence can lead to an unwanted side effect: the loss of a sense of our own presence. Not only is our pain invisible, but we may feel at least partially invisible ourselves, since we simply aren't expressing and communicating the truth of our experience.

Being from New England, I was raised on stoicism. It was considered selfish to complain or ask for help, so I was very reluctant to describe or discuss my pain with anyone. I tended toward understatement in order not to have a fuss made over me.

I think I was also unconsciously conforming to the lingering cultural and societal role of women as primarily nurturers and caretakers who are reluctant to ask for anything for ourselves.

This is also true for anyone taught not to draw attention to themselves, or those who were punished or disapproved of for needing help. For example, many young men have been shamed or punished for showing feelings or pain and for not being tough enough.

In addition, I worried that I was burdensome to others and disliked talking about how I was doing, since I could find nothing much good to report. I didn't want to be a negative person, and I didn't want people to feel bad for me.

I also didn't want to have to explain myself constantly, so I avoided talking about the pain I was in and pretended things were better than they really were.

All of this led to a reluctance to speak about what was really going on for me, a kind of silencing of the self. I expressed a very small part of me outwardly, while the vaster me lived in deep silence within an impermeable bubble suffused with the noise of pain.

This tendency toward silence kept me from fully and clearly delineating my symptoms at times when it would have been better to be very direct and clear about them. This felt like living in a surreal world, since others could see my body but not my pain.

I quickly began to see that most people are fairly uncomfortable with pain. I think that not only do they feel bad for the person who is suffering, but they also feel powerless to help. I would never ask anyone to heal me, but for many caring people the presence of someone in pain seems to require them to at least *try* to heal, fix, or advise.

Furthermore, my continued pain seemed to point out the fact that they were unable to really help me, to mend what was wrong. It seemed to highlight their inability to make it all better.

Antidotes to Invisibility and Silence

Share Your Feelings

While in pain, you will necessarily be silent about it a great deal of the time in order not to wear out, frighten, or worry others. However, when your silence leads to feelings of invisibility, unreality, or disconnection, it is important to find someone with whom you can safely share the true extent of your challenges and feelings.

This takes a special person who can be comfortable with strong feelings. Ask a good friend or family member if they will just listen and not offer advice or try to make you feel differently for the time being.

If a pain support group is available near you and you can get to it, that can be a safe outlet for feelings, since you know that people there will understand what you're going through. If you are a member of a church, temple, or other spiritual organization, talking with your minister, rabbi, or spiritual teacher can be another good option.

Seek Out a Reliable Professional

Talking about pain can be relieving, but it can also bring up other emotions that you haven't yet faced.

I always hated talking about the extent of my symptoms and pain to various doctors because afterward I felt sad, discouraged, and somewhat depressed. I was going through my days carrying on as best I could, and I found it easier to try not to think about my life or feel the emotions that were right under the surface.

I think we do this often in an effort to make it easier on ourselves and others, but it is also important to create a space for ourselves to feel the disappointment, frustration, and sadness that accompany our continuous pain, so these feelings don't just pool up inside of us.

If you think that your emotions are too strong to express to a friend or family member, or you feel that your emotions are overwhelming or unending, you may want to work through them with a professional therapist.

It can be immensely helpful to visit a professional person who can hear what you have to say without your feeling like you have to be positive about it. It helps release some of the pent-up grief and anger over the situation. It can also be a great relief to know you are going to be seeing that person repeatedly over time. If a therapist is not financially feasible, look into nonprofit organizations in your area that may provide mental and emotional health services for those in pain for a reduced fee or no fee.

Keep a Journal

It can also help to write your feelings in a journal, if writing is an option available to you in your condition. This is the place you can be wholly uncensored and raw if you need to. You can complain and rant and carry on about anything and everything that bothers you, and you don't have to worry about hurting anyone else's feelings or having them worry about your mental health.

In a journal you can let it all out. You can also do a lot of good thinking through writing, mulling over what you may be learning from this whole experience and what wisdom you can discover for your life and share with others.

Talk to an Animal

Animals are not to be underrated as agents of solace and healing. If you have a cat, dog, bird, guinea pig, or even a fish, use them as an extra ear.

Animals can be very patient (especially when they are asleep). You may feel foolish at first, but it is amazingly helpful to unburden yourself of your unspeakable feelings, angers, blames, and shames to at least one living being who will not contradict, edit, or counsel, but will hear you out and love you all the same.

SUMMARY

- Share your feelings.
- Seek out a reliable professional.
- Keep a journal.
- Talk to an animal.

12 Physical and Emotional Exhaustion

Being in pain is exhausting physically and emotionally. It wears us out because our bodies are working overtime to heal, because we are busy pushing against the experience of pain, because we are worrying about the future, because we can't sleep well, and because we are constricting the painful area and holding our breath.

Instead of resting peacefully so we can heal, we're going through things in our minds over and over again, trying to make sense of it all, trying to come to good decisions about medical options, and trying to plan how we'll handle all possible contingencies. Instead of getting a good night's sleep, we are restless due to pain and worry, and we wake up tired and foggy-brained.

When the mind twirls and whirls around about the illness or injury, about what it all means and why it is happening, it is very tiring. Because this kind of thinking is mostly rehashing, it is not very productive and takes a lot of energy. It drains rather than sustains.

When we are in pain, we naturally pull inward and constrict the area that is in pain in an effort to stop or at least lessen the pain sensations. By tensing the area in pain we restrict the necessary movement and flow in the body that brings healing.

We also may make a habit of holding the breath because it hurts to move and it hurts to feel. Holding the breath makes us feel like we're in control, but it is also fatiguing and contributes to the overall experience of being tired and worn-out.

All of these reactions are exhausting, particularly because they do not bring good results. They are an attempt to stop what is happening in our bodies rather than to trust the body to flow with and through the pain and, in that flow, to begin to heal.

We tighten when we might instead allow ourselves to let go of some of that holding and, bit by bit, relax into healing, trusting that pain is actually part of the healing process.

Antidotes to Physical and Emotional Exhaustion

Breathe

Pay attention to when and how you are holding your breath or using your breath to push against pain.

Make it a habit to notice how you are breathing and then to consciously release your breath at various times throughout the day.

Imagine your breath is your life force, the force for healing moving through your body, especially in the painful areas, and allow it to flow more freely.

Try to allow your breath to deepen if you are able to without raising pain levels. Take slower, longer breaths when you can (see "Exercise: Releasing Breath," page 106).

Relax Constricted Areas

When I realized I was tensing my body to try to not feel the pain or to keep it in one spot, I decided to experiment with deliberately relaxing the areas that hurt most in my body.

Sometimes it was impossible to relax the areas that were really shrieking in pain, so I focused on softening the areas *around* the pain instead (see "Exercise: Unlocking Contraction," page 110).

Give Rest a Rhythm

Most of us are aware that we need to rest more when we're in pain, but sometimes deep rest is hard to come by because pain won't allow it.

What worked for me was (a) to decide that rest was more important for healing than almost anything else I could do, (b) to pay attention to the quality of rest I was getting and notice what worked and what didn't, and (c) to give rest a rhythm.

The body requires more rest than usual in order to heal, yet we're often getting very little sleep at night due to pain-induced insomnia, so it helps to create many small rest periods during the day. This worked better for me than suffering through a whole night of tossing and turning and then trying to be up and about most of the next day.

Giving rest a rhythm requires noticing what times of day you rest more easily. We are so used to overriding the body's signals for rest during our usual workday life that we can continue that pattern when we're trying to heal.

When you're in pain, it takes more energy than you realize to do just about anything, including reading, watching a movie, or talking with others. Don't wait to feel like you need to rest.

Even if you think you won't sleep, map out half a dozen times during the day for complete rest. Sit or lie and breathe calmly. These rest periods are extremely important and helpful.

If you are working while in pain, this can be tricky, but jobs allow breaks that you can use for this. You can often simply stop, close your eyes, take a few calming breaths, and deliberately relax. (Go into the restroom to do this, if you need to.)

If you can't sleep through the night, get up and make a cup of herbal tea or sit up and read and then go back to bed. I usually found that this worked better than tossing around for hours.

I found that I slept best from 4:30 to 8:30 AM, and just knowing that this was my rhythm made it easier for me. I also found I could sleep for a half hour or so in the mid-afternoon, and I planned my schedule accordingly and made it as regular as I could.

Don't forget to use nature to help restore your body. Sitting outside and dozing in the warm sun can be more restful than lying inside on a bed or couch. Make a comfortable spot outside if you can, and lie on your balcony or patio if you have one; let the fresh air act as a restful restorative.

Reduce Inflammation

Recent research suggests that much of the pain in our bodies is due to inflammation. Researching anti-inflammatory diets and following that advice helped reduce my pain level as well as increase my sense of well-being and the overall energy level in my body. This includes cutting out or at least limiting caffeine, alcohol, and sugar among other inflammatory substances.

I also avoid media that cause stress and tightening in the body. I use simple ways to help my body and emotions relax, such as drinking herbal teas, listening to quiet music, and reading enjoyable, light books.

Cumulatively, these small changes do a great deal to help reduce overall body pain.

Stop Asking Why

Going around and around in your head about why this has happened or what you could have done to prevent it, or worrying about not healing faster, is unproductive and emotionally exhausting.

I did a lot of this at first, but I eventually stopped asking the unanswerable questions *Why me? Why now?* I accepted that I was in the situation I was in and that fretting about it was not conducive to ending it faster. I decided to ease up on myself and stop demanding healing from myself and from my body. I realized that the most positive approach was to take all the time my body needed to heal, and not try to rush what simply couldn't be rushed. This relieved me of a lot of unhelpful anxiety and allowed me to relax more and get deeper, more complete rest.

SUMMARY

- Breathe.
- Relax constricted areas.
- Give rest a rhythm.
- Reduce inflammation.
- Stop asking why.

13   Sadness and Loss

When we're in severe or chronic pain, our normal life is not available to us in the way it used to be. It isn't the same as going on vacation, or moving to another town, both of which we consciously choose as enjoyable breaks from the everyday.

Instead, living in pain feels like being taken *out* of life. Our normal life recedes to a distance at the same time that the feeling world of pain becomes incredibly close, immediate, and demanding. Pain *becomes* our experience of life.

We may still be physically present, but most of our energy and attention is busy elsewhere, trying to attend to pain or keep it at bay or heal our bodies or worry about how it will all work out. We simply aren't available to, or involved with, everyday life in the same way, and it does not feel like everyday life is available to us either.

The time spent in pain can feel like lost time. This is particularly sad when you cannot attend or participate in important events, or when you must do so in your aura of pain. Even when you can participate, pain limits your enjoyment and leaves you with a feeling of not having been entirely present.

My time in pain has been particularly heartbreaking for me in terms of being a parent. I have been unable to participate and contribute in many of the ways I have wanted to, and I have felt an immense sense of loss.

I used to be a world traveler and very active, so I had planned to travel and go backpacking and camping with my son. When I was injured, I was in the process of teaching him to swim, and we'd gotten our bicycles tuned up for some long rides. All that went out the window.

In addition to that loss, I was no longer able to work, which meant that I lost not only my ability to support myself financially but my hopes and dreams for my career. This was also true of my avocations. I had begun a series of watercolor paintings and had some interest from art galleries, but my injury forced me to put that project on the shelf indefinitely.

Anyone who experiences pain over time has stories like these. You feel sadness and loss not only for the time and experiences that are eaten up by pain but also for lost dreams and goals, as if your connection to the future is being consumed by pain as well.

Antidotes to Sadness and Loss

View Pain as a Landscape You're Passing Through

Since pain feels all-encompassing while you are experiencing it (I think that's why we describe it as being *in* pain), it's easy to lose the ability to imagine anything else. It can be really difficult to remember what it feels like *not* to be in pain.

One day I woke up and realized I didn't have a sense of a personal future anymore. I had simply stopped dreaming because it seemed like my life was just going to be an endless stream of days in pain. So I started to think of pain as a landscape that had edges. It had a beginning, therefore it must have an end. Somewhere.

The landscape was nasty, ugly, and burned-out, but it was only a landscape, a place I was walking *through*, not the entire world. I told myself that I would eventually reach other landscapes. I was just passing through this one.

This helped restore a sense of having a future. Soon after creating and working with the various exercises and antidotes in this book, I began noticing more green on the horizon of my pain landscape, buds on the blackened branches, and a rustle here and there in the bracken denoting small things coming back to life.

Look for the Gold in the Ashes

I have found it very difficult to deal with the sense of loss I feel due to the amount of time I have spent in pain. I have had to reframe the way I see those years. Instead of representing life lost, they represent a different *kind* of life, equally valuable, even if I couldn't yet completely see how.

When I went in search of the gold in all the ashes, I realized that my son had learned some valuable life lessons through my painful condition.

He learned to think about someone else's well-being other than just his own and not to take life and health for granted. He learned that he was important and his contribution really counted, since I needed his help daily to do basic household tasks.

Living in pain can give you valuable insights. You will be bringing back a greater awareness of what others suffer and greater compassion for others. You can develop a fuller sense of gratitude for all the relationships in your life and a deeper appreciation for your body.

If you decide to delve more fully into the emotional aspects of being in pain, you may find expression for difficult feelings that need to move on. Working through these emotional aspects can allow a greater sense of freedom in life, even while you are still in pain.

Choose New Meaning

And, finally, when it feels like life in pain is meaningless, I remind myself that it is I who choose the meaning of my life.

I can decide that I have wasted or lost the years I have been in pain, or I can choose to see them as years with a different *kind* of meaning.

Through my time spent with pain, I have, sometimes begrudgingly, learned a great deal about what it is to be a human being and how to find a deeper sense of an overreaching arc and flow in my life and the value of life's natural vicissitudes.

SUMMARY

- Pain is a landscape you're passing through.
- Look for the gold in the ashes.
- Choose new meaning.

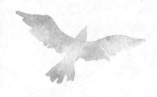

PART 3

Meditative Approaches
to Physical Pain

14   Discovering Pain's Purpose

In the Western allopathic medical world, physical pain is treated almost entirely from a material standpoint.

In our highly technological and sometimes formulaic culture, we think we will fix our pains if we can just land on the right approach from a confusing and often contradictory variety of programs, pharmaceuticals, cures, and techniques: Pop these pills, take this yoga class, read this book, start eating this, stop eating that, get off the couch, relax more, get out more. We tend to treat pain solely with physically based remedies or to mask it with chemical inhibitors.

Our doctor usually asks us where and how it hurts, and we are encouraged to describe the pain only as it is manifesting in the body. It is a rare Western-trained doctor who asks the patient how they feel *about* the pain emotionally, what was going on in their life just before the onset of pain, or a myriad of other inquiries into the patient's emotional, psychological, and spiritual state of being.

One of the reasons that we usually don't treat physical pain with anything more than physical remedies is that, most obviously, it is experienced in and through the body. Physical pain is so overwhelming for the sufferer that it appears to point only to itself. This seems logical. Yet, while we do live in a physical body, we also consist of a mind and emotions, and many believe we have a spirit or soul as well.

Despite the lack of clear boundaries between these aspects of the self, we have developed different therapeutic approaches, models, and remedies for each, as if each could be addressed uniquely and apart from its impact or reliance on the others.

Consequently, the prevailing medical language refers to the body as a thing, an object, an impersonal lump of flesh. Its physicality is somehow unrelated to the parts of us we can't see, but which we may, nevertheless, consider the essence of who we really are. The body is inexplicably, but fundamentally, treated as separate from the inner *us*.

Similarly, we talk about our conditions, our pain, and the organs and systems of our bodies as if each had a life of its own as a disparate entity.

We name our conditions and refer to them by those names, as if we have been invaded by an outside force that remains distinct and separate even though it is completely interwoven with our bodies, our thoughts, and our feelings. Our condition literally lives in us and with us, yet we speak of it as something that could be pointed to and catalogued and extracted.

Although much has been written in recent years about body/mind/spirit integration, particularly in connection with the rising popularity of traditional Asian medicine and acupuncture, the Western medical approach is only beginning to adopt the concept that treatments need to include and address the whole person. Ultimately, therefore, while hugely beneficial in many cases, our scientific approach to life and to health has taught us to compartmentalize our bodies, our lives, our selves, and our pain.

Meanwhile, a growing number of people are not finding relief from pain medications or medical treatments of any kind, and doctors are finding a growing number of painful conditions, such as fibromyalgia and thoracic outlet syndrome, that are difficult to diagnose clearly or treat successfully.

Additionally, we have been conditioned by our culture to keep going no matter what. We are not taught to listen to the body, or to our emotions and feeling states as they relate to the body, and certainly not to listen to or honor pain. We override the body's signals routinely by working too many long days, by overeating or undereating, and by using various substances to feel energized when we're exhausted or to calm down when we're hyper.

In a society driven by schedules and fairly rigid work and educational structures, it's probably a natural consequence that we would develop a medical system that makes getting back on track as soon as possible one of its top priorities. Nothing seems to be wrong with that on the surface, but what if, by doing that, we are sidestepping a significant purpose within the process of healing?

What might be the consequences of ignoring the body's signals, its method of communication? What if, instead of killing, or utterly eradicating, pain with pharmaceuticals, we used medications primarily to reduce pain to a manageable level, so that we can still hear what the body means to tell us in the language of pain? By not honoring the body's inner timetable and how it relates to our whole self, we might be derailing a deeper meaning held within the pain. If so, then it is possible that this inner purpose unfolds only when we respect it and give it the time and attention it seems to be asking for.

⚜

Dear Pain,

I really want you to go away. You have been an unwelcome guest in my life for too long. I'm hoping that if I try to understand you, you will be satisfied and leave. But the truth is, I really don't want to know you. I don't want to have to know you.

You are like an unwelcome stranger who shows up at my house needing a meal. I make him a sandwich and want to send him on his way, but he won't leave. He is smelly and strange, his disheveled appearance is alarming, he mumbles to himself, and I realize he's crazy and unreachable and I don't want to have to touch him. I don't want to have to know him. And I certainly don't want him to touch me.

I know I'm supposed to feel differently, to have compassion, but I don't want to have to do more. I'm praying he doesn't sit on the couch, and could he just take twenty dollars and leave? You are like that stranger, Pain. I want the minimum interaction with you so you will be satisfied and go away.

15 The Body Made Wrong

When I was unable to heal after a long period of time, I became frustrated and distressed. I hated the situation I was in, and I worried that people might think I wasn't trying hard enough to recover, since there was no discernible improvement.

In fact, things seemed to keep getting worse. I needed my body to respond. I needed it to mend. It was betraying me.

Deep down, though, a nagging feeling suggested that somehow I might be betraying my body. After months and months of pushing toward healing with no positive results, I had to wonder how I could create true health if I was constantly peeved and frustrated with myself, my body, and the pain in my body.

During my long days with nothing to do, I started to wonder how I could better understand the genuine needs not only of my body but of my emotions, mind, and spirit.

My physical symptoms and condition were intrinsically interwoven not only with one another but with my current experience of myself and of life. None of them could be completely separated out.

Till then, I had been reacting against pain and attempting to push it out of me. For the most part, I felt abandoned by life and by whatever divine force there was in the universe. I felt disconnected from most of my friends. Pain was the strongest reality and the most insistent presence in my life. Why couldn't I make it go away? What good could its continued presence possibly be doing?

I thought that I simply had to find the *right* healing modality, the *right* doctor, the *right* therapist, or the *right* regimen.

But what did I really know about how the body heals? What was it trying to communicate *through* the pain? In how many different ways was I simply refusing to acknowledge its messages?

When I looked at the situation from a different perspective, however, it seemed to me that my body wasn't just responding *with* pain; it was also *experiencing* it. My body was suffering the pain with me. We were in it together.

While it sometimes felt like it was working against me because it was producing the pain, my body was actually doing its utter best to heal and, ultimately, help me feel better.

Understanding that my body was not the enemy, I also came to realize that pain was not the enemy either. The sensation of pain, while unpleasant to the extreme, was actually the body's signal that it was making every effort to heal.

My body was my only ticket to planet Earth, and if I wanted to stick around, I would have to discover what it required to make it well and whole again. One of the initial movements toward healing my body, then, was to change my attitude toward it and toward its pain messages.

I thought I was giving pain the attention it truly deserved by trying to be rid of it. That's what you do with pain; you try to end it. I wasn't tuning in to the pain itself as itself, which seemed like a very bad idea.

Turning toward pain in an attempt to notice it more fully seemed like it would only make things worse.

❧

Dear Pain,

Despite your jarring quality, I try to relax, take deep breaths. The deeper the breath, the more it hurts. I adjust back to shallower breaths.

Trying to hold my spine erect in meditation posture annoys you to no end, and you soon begin shooting long darts into my neck that twang mercilessly and resonate fully before subsiding and making way for the next.

This is obviously not working.

So I stop, I listen.

Perhaps if I give you the attention you demand (deserve?), you will be satisfied for a while and give me some respite.

My hope is that giving you respectful attention will lead to healing. If you are allowed to have your say to a truly attentive audience (me), you will have fulfilled your purpose, satisfied your needs to be seen and heard, and like a little kid to whom the adult finally leans over and gives their undivided attention, you will be satisfied and leave me alone.

I sit and listen, your insistent sounds amplified by my focus, but it seems I do not speak your language.

I ask you questions about who you might be, what you might represent, but you just blare atonally.

Like a very nasty gremlin, you repay my vigilance with arrows and insults. I cannot distinguish any vocabulary that I recognize.

16   Finding a New Approach

After years of unsuccessful efforts to diminish, expel, erad-icate, and overcome the pain in my body, I wondered if the pain sensations might be a voice for not only the body but other levels of the self as well.

I understood that, while pain felt strong and overbear-ing and it absolutely dominated my attention, it was not necessarily an adversarial power. It was a reaction.

Pain accompanied me in a most unpleasant manner, but it was a signal to be received and decoded, not a foe to be fought and annihilated. Allowing it space to express itself seemed counterproductive; still, I began to wonder what could happen if I began to *respect and honor* my pain.

While it seemed to be the demanding dictator of my life because it was so loud and insistent, I understood that it was also a messenger. It was the effect of something. It signaled, it warned, it annoyed, but that was part of its purpose.

Pain was fulfilling its mission.

I finally realized that I wasn't going to be able to even start the process of true healing until I had achieved a deeper level of trust with the inner wisdom that was running my physical system.

It seemed that it had a road map to health in its own language that I wasn't privy to or hadn't bothered to learn. It occurred to me that I might even be delaying my recovery and prolonging my time in pain by trying to hurry things along at my own preferred pace.

What if I needed to back down, relax, enter a state of calm, and learn to listen to the innate wisdom of my body and inner self through the code expressed as pain?

What if I did something radical and sort of uncovered my ears and eyes and really tried to see and hear what this pain in my body was trying to say to me, instead of constantly attempting to overcome it, close it down, and basically shut it up?

What possibilities for healing might open up if I began to relate to it as part of an interconnected system, *me*, the whole me, and began to tune in to the ways it was communicating?

How, then, could I find a way to be in a different relationship with pain so that I was no longer utterly beholden to it, but without treating it as an adversary? I asked myself, if pain were *my* voice, what might I be trying to tell myself?

Since nothing I was doing to stop it was working, I decided to open up to the possibility of healing through meeting pain where and how it wanted to be met.

What this meant, I wasn't exactly sure, but it occurred to me that the degree to which I could listen to and interact positively with the pain that was living in my body might be the degree to which I could heal.

It goes against our current ideas of health to let pain be felt fully and to respond to it as an agent of healing. Yet, despite our usual rejection of anything painful, I felt that maybe there was untapped wisdom to be found within the experience of pain itself.

Perhaps the manifestation of the profoundest healing included an understanding that pain sensations may be more than just a physical reaction; they may include an expression of deeper levels of the self as well.

The answer, for me, lay in finding a way to understand pain from a more holistic perspective and to see it from a positive standpoint.

This meant seeing myself not as a helpless victim but as someone on a journey. It meant looking at pain as a signpost and a guide, not a problem to be overcome.

It meant letting go of the mentality that I was at the mercy of my condition and my circumstances. Instead of seeing pain as an invader and a curse, I could imagine it as part of something that was trying to heal itself in my life and, somehow, *through* my life — an expression of something that wanted to make me whole.

⊹

Dear Pain,

So, here's what I haven't allowed before because I feared, like my fantasy of the unbathed odiferous stranger, that if I gave you that much space, you would want the whole house. Could I trust the stranger to take only what he really needed if I opened my house to him? Is that the right thing to do?

So I fear you're like that, Pain. I fear you are insatiable.

You sure seem to be — you show up in my face every hour of every day demanding attention. But if I give you more attention, won't you take even more from me? What if I dared to give you a voice and listened to what you had to say? Could I risk giving you that much power? That much room?

I7   Communicating with Pain

Once I realized that pain was not going to be leaving my body anytime soon and that I simply didn't understand its purpose, I decided to meet it face-to-face, so to speak. I wondered what pain would look like if it appeared in front of me for the purposes of a dialogue.

This intrigued me. If pain took form, I could ask it questions. I could see the meaning it held in the form it took. I could see it as something with boundaries rather than an all-consuming reality.

From that point on, I began to dream up new avenues of dialogue with pain in order to understand how it connected with and was interwoven through both the physical and the nonphysical layers of the self. I created ways to interact with pain differently, to establish a new kind of relationship with it and, ultimately, with myself.

I began by getting quiet. I asked pain questions. I wrote letters to pain. I played with the idea of pain as a messenger, a character, a force for good. I wanted to know what pain had to do with me and how it expressed as me and through me. I turned my ideas about pain on their head.

The results were very encouraging. Pain did not leave my body all at once or even completely. But it began to get quieter, less intense. It reacted like a wounded creature that finally felt safe or an angry child soothed. It stepped down, so to speak. It relaxed.

And the most important thing I found was that I needed to allow pain to be what it was, *as* it was, before I could expect it to move on.

I understood that, in some strange way, it felt heard and respected. That seemed like an absolutely key understanding. Pain was something in me that, perhaps inexplicably, but in a very real way, *needed a different kind of attention.*

It occurred to me that pain wouldn't leave until I recognized its purpose and said yes to whatever it needed to give me, tell me, or show me. This allowed me to see pain as something that offered me a gift, strange as it might be, and the opportunity to consciously choose to accept this gift.

I began experimenting with how I related to the pain in my body and how that relationship affected all the other relationships in my life, including my relationship with myself.

To me, pain seemed very much like a little child pulling on a pant leg and whining. You keep telling the child to stop and be quiet but they only get more upset. Finally, you take a breath, squat down, look the child in the eyes, and calmly ask, *What would you like to tell me?*

I'm not saying that your pain is a child stuck inside of you (or maybe that's not so far off the mark), but something is calling to be noticed and responded to, and most of us simply try to make it stop. I discovered that when I decided to give pain all the time it needs, turn toward it, so to speak, and pay attention to it, it almost immediately began to relax and release.

I wanted to find out if the gift or the message was from pain itself, from life, from my body, or from me to me. Or maybe it didn't matter; it was all really the same thing.

Working with these creative avenues helped me to stop trying to attack my pain and, instead, to find ways to be with my experience differently and, ultimately, more positively.

They opened the door to listening to, hearing, and responding to pain in ways that were more conducive to deep healing.

⁕

Dear Pain,

Ignoring you altogether doesn't work because it means I overextend myself and that makes my condition worse, which gives you headway to get even louder and more insistent.

Meditation seems like an obvious choice to create the relaxation so necessary to physical healing, but as soon as I quiet everything else in order to sit in silence, there you are. An empty stage.

You take that as an opportunity to create strident improvisations on your terrible horns. Pains I haven't felt all day in my feet and fingers now appear in full living stereo. Did my head hurt this much five minutes ago? Even my butt is tingling and burning.

Okay. I acknowledge you, Pain. I go into you and try to relax into being the captive audience I really am, like an exhausted parent who patiently listens attentively, even lovingly, to the screeching tones of someone else's children in a musical concert.

18 Soothing the Wounded Animal

One of the most useful metaphors I have found in working with pain is to imagine it as a wild animal, injured and alone.

What would we do if we found a wild animal shivering, scared, hurt, and bleeding in our home? We certainly wouldn't want to rush right up and try to touch it or move it because we'd most probably frighten it more, and the animal would feel threatened and possibly bite us.

What would be our reaction to this situation? Would we get angry with the animal for ruining our home and shout at it? Would we try to find a way to forcibly remove it? Would we leave the room, close it up tight, and lock the door?

Interestingly, this situation is an apt metaphor for the way we are with our pain. We treat it as an unwelcome invader. We want it out of our body as fast as possible. We try to find the Animal Control person to have it removed.

Yet it refuses to budge. We try to ignore it, but it's in there growling or howling or whimpering all the time. What do we do?

If we decide to help the wounded animal in our house, we might try opening the door very slowly and enter the room a little ways or just stand in the doorway. We would let the animal know we're there and we're not going to hurt it. We would let it get used to our presence. We would look at it with kindness and just *be* with it. We might sit down so we don't appear threatening.

As we do this, the animal begins to look differently to us, and it looks at us differently. We stop seeing only its fangs and claws and notice the caked blood and dirt on its fur, that it needs care, and how frightened and alone it is. We begin to have compassion for it. We speak soothingly to it.

We lose our concern with getting rid of it as we become more interested in helping and taking care of it. Instead of trying to delete it from our experience, we decide to include it. After all, it's already in the house.

We may move a little closer and notice its reaction. We see how it gets used to our presence, how our caring attention allows it to relax a little.

Over time, it lets us get close enough to clean its wounds and care for it. We see how it relaxes under our gentle touch. We notice that it is a beautiful animal beneath the encrusted blood and matted fur.

As we befriend the animal, as it allows us to care for it, we find that underneath the hurt there is a potential ally; a fox, a dog, a wild cat, or a majestic bird of prey. It holds an energy and an intelligence that is available to enrich our lives.

Possibly it is the energy of something we hid away long ago or of something or someone forgotten from childhood. Perhaps it is a part of our forgotten selves.

We want to approach our pain in much the same way we would approach this wounded animal. With care, with soothing words.

We want to create trust and establish a relationship based on respect, even if, at first, it's from a wary distance. We allow the relationship to become less mistrustful and more open over time.

We accept that pain is already in our house and isn't leaving through force. We learn to treat it as if, underneath the fangs and the claws, it carries a valuable gift for our lives, something we need to know, to understand, to be with, to accept, and to grow into.

The pain is not the gift, but it points to the gift. It is a signal that the wounded animal has arrived and needs our respectful and caring attention.

Our refusal to accept the pain, the presence of the wounded animal inside ourselves, creates a situation in which the messenger must wait and wait for us to pay it the attention it requires. It becomes locked up in a room in our house, so to speak, waiting for us to discover its purpose.

Pain that refuses to leave, that becomes chronic, may be at least partially related to our misunderstanding of pain's purposes, our inability to see and accept the gifts that pain brings.

Our reluctance to find the gifts in our pain may be a

product of ignorance, of course. We have been taught all our lives that pain is bad, and our natural reaction is to avoid it.

Another aspect of our reluctance to be with the wounded animal may also be because, in order to help the animal, to become its caretaker, we must change our perspective. We must alter our perspective from seeing the animal as a dangerous nuisance to seeing it as a potential friend and ally.

Because pain is part of our experience of ourselves right now, this means that healing requires that we also change our perspective on ourselves, at the very least, and very possibly on life, on others, on the past, and on the future.

We must shift something within us in order to receive the gift that pain brings. We must approach a painful aspect of ourselves and soothe it, accept it, respect it, and allow it to unfold its message and its story.

In the eleven simple meditative exercises that follow, I invite you to establish a new relationship and dialogue with pain.

19 Introduction to Meditative Exercises

While medications and procedures work on our physicality to try to cure whatever ails us through traditional medical means, the eleven meditative exercises that follow honor the inner world of pain and the inner relationships pain establishes within and between the body and the self.

Through them, we set up lines of communication with pain as an energy, a personality, and a messenger. In some, we step back to see pain from a distance, and in others, we draw in closer to understand it even more intimately.

By gaining some distance, we can see that pain is not the totality of who we are. By stepping in closer, we see how it expresses itself in our bodies using metaphor and imagination.

By creating a new relationship with pain, opening up lines of communication, and understanding pain's inner purposes and messages, we can begin to loosen the hold it has on our bodies, thereby easing symptoms and shortening its stay.

Doing these short meditative exercises helps release anxiety and increase our overall emotional and physical well-being.

After a brief explanation, each exercise provides a direct experience of the concepts. If you do not feel up to doing the meditative exercises at this time, please finish reading through them anyway, since they introduce many helpful approaches and insights.

Each exercise is relatively short. I recommend working with them in a progression, as they build on one another. Each can be done any number of times.

Since some of these exercises bring directed awareness to the sensations of physical pain, use your discretion in deciding when it is time to rest.

Through working this way, I discovered that while I was putting my directed attention on pain, it did briefly seem more intense, but paradoxically, this respectful attention led to greater relief and release both over the duration of each exercise and as I worked with them repeatedly over time.

Be kind to yourself as you experiment with relating to your pain in new ways. Take it slow with frequent rests, and talk to others about your feelings when you can.

Each exercise is preceded by a ✒ symbol.

20   Releasing Breath

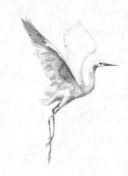

One of the first things we do when we experience pain is draw in a sharp breath and hold it to try to stop the painful sensation.

Holding the breath puts us in a kind of suspended animation where it seems we don't have to feel. When we resume breathing, it's usually shallow and light, punctuated by sharp intakes or panting, and then we periodically hold the breath again.

We avoid breathing with or into the pain; we try to use our breath to eject pain from the body or to create a wall of breath that the pain can't get past.

Holding the breath obviously impedes the flow of oxygen into the bloodstream; it also tightens muscles and increases the overall constriction in the body. If we continuously impede our natural breathing process, it has a deleterious effect on our health and our healing possibilities.

Once I noticed my habit of holding or restricting my breath, I began to consciously try to release it and to breathe more fully and calmly. The more I could breathe into and with my pain rather than against it, the better I felt.

✒ EXERCISE: RELEASING BREATH

1. Notice How You Are Breathing

This is a very simple exercise, but extremely important. From time to time throughout your day, put attention on how you are breathing.

Are you holding your breath, panting shallowly, or taking short, erratic breaths? Are you pushing against the pain with your breath, or trying to avoid feelings (physical and emotional) by not breathing fully?

2. Release Your Breath

If you notice that you have a habit of holding your breath, simply relax, breath in, and exhale calmly. This breath does not have to be particularly deep or slow; just start with allowing it to be a little freer and a little calmer.

See if you can release the breath and use it less and less as a wall for holding back the pain.

If you are panting, experiment with slowing your breath into a more natural rhythm. Alternatively, experiment with panting more, even speeding it up some (without hyperventilating), and then releasing it.

3. Notice How Breath Affects Your Pain Levels

Notice how placing attention on your breath and allowing it to flow more easily affects your pain levels. Pain may go up at first or stay the same, but over time, it should reduce bit by bit as you allow your breath to move through your body with less restriction.

Do this exercise again and again, putting awareness on your breath and simply allowing it to restore itself to its natural flow as much as possible.

EXERCISE REVIEW: RELEASING BREATH

1. Notice how you are breathing.
2. Release your breath.
3. Notice how breath affects your pain levels.

21   Unlocking Contraction

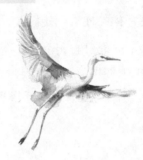

Pain is usually accompanied by contraction in the body. Our bodies become tighter and more held in, similar to how we withdraw suddenly from something too hot or too dangerous.

The problem with this response is that, when in pain, we are not withdrawing from something external; we are withdrawing from something we are experiencing on the inside. We are effectively trying to pull ourselves away from the part of us that is in pain.

Since this is physically impossible, over time it tends to create increased tension and contraction in the body. In an effort to avoid the pain, we create a kind of lockdown effect, tightening the painful area in order to isolate it from our experience and the rest of the body. Being in this lockdown state is usually also accompanied by withheld or restricted breathing.

As we work to loosen up the breath and allow it to flow, we also want to allow the body to decompress, so to speak.

Pulling away from the pain or clamping down in that area in order to keep the pain in one place or in an attempt to minimize it actually makes it worse. When we attempt to keep the pain from moving or growing, we are effectively holding it in place.

Usually, we don't want to give pain anything; we just want it to go away. But, paradoxically, giving pain breath and space begins to relax the area in pain and the body around the pain, which provides some relief.

At first it may feel like the pain is getting worse because you are allowing yourself to notice it more fully, but then, as you stay with the exercise, you should notice it easing up.

✒ EXERCISE: UNLOCKING CONTRACTION

1. Notice the Contraction

Notice how your body feels pulled in, contracted, compressed, or tight in and around the areas in pain. Just pay attention to what this feels like.

Notice how small you are trying to make the painful area, and notice if your breathing stops as soon as you tune in to your pain.

2. Imagine Space Around the Pain

Feel the contracted area of pain, and then notice that there is space around the pain that is pain-free.

If your pain is intense, you may find that this pain-free space starts at a distance from the pain. It's possible that the only area not in pain may be experienced as outside of the body.

Let your attention go back and forth gently from the painful contraction to the pain-free space, then to the pain, then to the space, back and forth slowly about four to six times.

3. Allow Your Pain More Space

This is going to seem counterintuitive, but begin to allow your pain to very gently relax into the space around it. Put your attention on the pain and the space around the pain at the same time.

Allow the pain to slowly expand into the space around it. You can imagine it unfurling, oozing, loosening, melting, or unclenching.

At first, it will seem like the pain is growing, but you will notice that if you can relax, trust, and avoid pulling it back in, it begins to gently dissipate as it relaxes into a larger and larger space.

Trust yourself to allow this to happen. The pain can always contract back again after this exercise if you need it to; don't worry.

4. Notice Any Changes in Your Pain

As the pain expands and relaxes into the space around it, notice if the intensity changes.

Is it less pointy, sharp, insistent, or intense, even for a split second? If it is, just notice that this means your pain can change, it can heal, it can release.

Don't expect it to happen all at once, but for now, just notice the new possibilities.

EXERCISE REVIEW: UNLOCKING CONTRACTION

1. Notice the contraction.
2. Imagine space around the pain.
3. Allow your pain more space.
4. Notice any changes in your pain.

22   Paying Attention to Pain

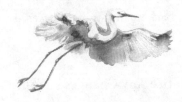

This may sound obvious or completely nonsensical, but we're going to practice really noticing the experience of pain.

You might immediately say: *How can I* not *notice it, when it's all I'm noticing!* But before you toss this book across the room, give it a moment and read further.

In this exercise, we're going to notice what happens when you calmly, respectfully, and graciously pay attention to your pain and just be with it.

Shifting from *resisting* pain to *allowing* the experience of pain can have a profound and immediate effect. Again, it's somewhat counterintuitive, but feeling the pain more fully can begin to relieve it.

EXERCISE: PAYING ATTENTION TO PAIN

1. Stop Resisting

Consciously choose to stop resisting your pain for the duration of this exercise. Relax your body around the pain as much as you can. Take some soft, calming breaths. Don't breathe too deeply if that increases your pain level.

2. Turn Toward Your Pain

In whatever way this makes sense to you, on the inside, consciously turn toward your pain and pay attention to it in a calm and receptive manner. Just acknowledge it, with no agenda of any kind. Greet it in whatever way you wish. (Say hello or give it a nod or a little pat.)

At first, your pain may seem to grow stronger and louder, just like a voice in a conversation that you suddenly tune in to, but this is an illusion. The pain is only as strong as it was a moment ago; you are just allowing yourself to notice what it really feels like.

3. Be with Your Pain without an Agenda

Be with your pain as you would be with a frightened child or a wild animal. Let it get used to you being this close, and let yourself get used to its nearness, as you continue to breathe calmly. Notice the pain sensation just as it is, for itself, and notice that it is not the totality of you. There is you looking at pain. There is the pain. You are together, but you are not the same thing.

4. Notice Everything about Your Pain

Notice everything you can about your pain. Does it feel rough, prickly, stabbing, aching, sharp, hot, frozen? Say the words that apply out loud: *Deep. Aching. Sharp. Stabbing.*

Notice its depth. Does it stay near the skin's surface or does it extend deeply into your body? Does it shift in any way as you pay attention to it?

Imagine what size and shape it is. Imagine its color, temperature, and texture. Say the applicable descriptive words out loud: *Red. Hot. Freezing. Numb. Icy. Prickly.* Notice any emotions that arise while you are paying attention to pain in this way.

5. Notice Any Changes

Spend as much time as you wish just being with your pain, noticing it for what it is, noticing all its attributes, and not trying to change it just yet. When you're done, simply return to normal consciousness. Notice any changes in the sensations and pain levels in your body.

EXERCISE REVIEW: PAYING ATTENTION TO PAIN

1. Stop resisting.
2. Turn toward your pain.
3. Be with your pain without an agenda.
4. Notice everything about your pain.
5. Notice any changes.

23 Shifting Your Relationship to Pain

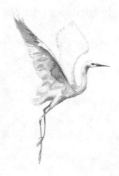

Much of this book works to find ways to shift our relationship with pain from one of negativity and animosity, or victimization and passivity, to one that is much more interactive and constructive.

It is very much about coming into rapport with the pain in your body and exploring approaches to pain management that respect and honor all aspects of the situation, including the difficult ones.

This exercise will help you consciously shift your relationship with pain in order to make room for greater healing and freedom of expression. It also looks at how your feelings about the pain in your body may reflect other relationships in your life, and you may have some moments of recognition.

As I have said, instead of trying to keep pain out in an effort to exclude it from your experience, you can choose to include it and create a more conscious relationship with it. Anything you forcefully exclude, you have no power over. Anything you willingly include, you can change.

✒ EXERCISE: SHIFTING YOUR RELATIONSHIP TO PAIN

1. Notice Your Relationship to Pain

What relationship do you have with pain right now? Is pain something you are still fighting, or are you a little more friendly toward it? How would you classify this relationship? Is it:

- tyrant/slave?
- mentor/student?
- torturer/captive?
- messenger/receiver?

2. Notice What Characterizes This Relationship

Is this relationship based on trust and open-mindedness or hatred and suspicion? Is it combative or friendly?

Are you noticing that distrust and resentment are beginning to shift toward acceptance and allowing?

3. Notice If This Mirrors Other Relationships

Does anything about your relationship with pain feel familiar?

Does it resemble any of your relationships with family members: mother, father, siblings, spouse, children?

How similar is it to your relationship to life? To your inner self?

4. Choose the Relationship You Prefer

What kind of relationship would you like to have with pain and why? What characterizes it? What would be most constructive, most restorative, most releasing, and most healing?

5. Begin Practicing This New Relationship

Begin to practice this new relationship to pain in your body. Decide to let go of whatever is keeping pain stuck, be it resentment, self-pity, blame, or any other contractive or downward-pulling emotion or feeling state.

If you find that your relationship with pain mirrors an existing relationship in your life, consider trying to shift both relationships in positive ways.

Let go of what you perceive needs to leave — attitudes, beliefs, resentments — and consciously choose to make room for something better for your body and for your life.

EXERCISE REVIEW: SHIFTING YOUR RELATIONSHIP TO PAIN

1. Notice your relationship to pain.
2. What characterizes this relationship?
3. Notice if this mirrors other relationships.
4. Choose the relationship you prefer.
5. Begin practicing this new relationship.

24 Loving the Places That Hurt

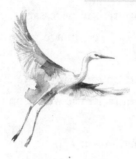

When trying to resist, kill, and eradicate my pain didn't work, I tried ignoring it and just living with it. But being stoic and putting up with it was only slightly better than fighting it. It made me less anxious because I was no longer in a battle with pain, but it did nothing to actually reduce the amount of pain I was experiencing.

I then decided to try something radical. I would do exactly the opposite of hating and trying to annihilate pain.

I decided to love it.

I couldn't fight pain, shouldn't fight it, so instead I would offer it softness, understanding, compassion, and inclusion, exactly what we are taught we must never do with pain.

Interestingly enough, it is also what we are taught we should never do with ourselves when we fail. Instead of offering ourselves softness and forgiveness, we are most often critical and harsh, telling ourselves to "get over it," "buck up," and "carry on."

We treat our pain in the same manner — as something unforgivable, unwanted, unnecessary, and with no redeeming qualities, like our self-image when we trip up badly in life.

We are as hard on our pain as we are on ourselves. And we are as hard on ourselves as we are on our pain. Interesting mirroring there.

This little meditation can be very helpful when done regularly. In it, you notice that pain is just part of your experience, not all of your experience. You are connecting your center of goodwill with the center of pain.

Notice any difference in your level of pain when you choose to send it positive feelings rather than negative. See what happens with the rest of your body when you send love and goodwill to your pain.

✒ EXERCISE: LOVING THE PLACES THAT HURT

1. Check In with Your Pain

Place a soft attention on your pain. If the pain is in more than one area of your body, choose one, perhaps the most acute, since it is the area that is literally crying out for the most attention.

Sit or lie and breathe quietly with the pain for a moment. Notice the circumference and shape of the pain. Send it a little hello.

2. Breathe into Your Heart

Now find the center of your heart, what you might think of as the center of your inner self.

Take a few calming breaths into your heart and notice that, despite the pain here or elsewhere, a capacity for peace, calm, and ease, no matter how minuscule, remains.

Take a few moments to notice these dual sensations, the calm and the pain, coexisting. They don't have to be mutually exclusive.

3. Send Kindness and Love to Your Pain

From your heart, send a feeling of goodwill to the painful area, no matter how small that feeling of goodwill is at the moment. Understand that the painful area is already doing its best to heal. Thank your body for its efforts to heal. Thank the pain for letting you know that something needs attention and healing.

Imagine love extending from your heart, your inner self, to encase the painful area very, very softly, like a mist.

You can also imagine a soft light, a peaceful meadow, a calm body of water, or any other soothing image that appeals to you gently encompassing the painful area.

Maintain a feeling of nonjudgmental kindness toward your pain and whatever it is trying to heal in your body and in your life.

4. Soothe Your Pain

Soothe the pain as if it is a child who has never had a kind word or a soft caress. Speak soothing words to it in your mind.

Notice if you have any resistance to being kind to yourself or to being kind to your pain.

EXERCISE REVIEW: LOVING THE PLACES THAT HURT

1. Check in with your pain.
2. Breathe into your heart.
3. Send kindness and love to your pain.
4. Soothe your pain.

25 Imaging Pain's Form

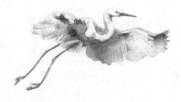

Art therapy is a time-honored approach to working with difficult emotions, and I used it to work with physical pain as well. I was able to do it only in a limited scope due to my condition, but the images, symbols, and metaphors that emerged were very revealing and helpful.

The simple act of nonverbal expression can be particularly healing. It helps ease the sense of feeling stuck, alone, misunderstood, or unable to describe or share the feelings that arise from living in pain.

This kind of image-making helps to bring forward what might be hidden, tends to help move stuck emotional energy, and can provide important insights.

It can connect you with long-buried emotions or tell a story you didn't realize you were holding within yourself.

I recommend inexpensive watercolor or poster paints for this exercise because it's usually easier to move a brush (rather than drawing with a pencil), and I feel that paint offers the most expressive potential in both the looseness of the medium and the use of color.

↵ EXERCISE: IMAGING PAIN'S FORM

1. Calm Your Mind and Body

With your art supplies at hand, take several slow inhales and exhales and consciously calm your mind and relax your body around the pain as much as you can.

2. Tune In to Your History with This Pain

Take a moment to tune in to your history with this pain.

Remember pain's beginning, however long ago, and how it led to what you are presently enduring. Imagine this as your pain story.

Notice that it has quieter times and more tumultuous times, almost like peaks and valleys on a timeline.

Feel into the whole form of your pain story in whatever way that makes sense to you.

3. Express from within Your Pain

Begin to paint with the intention of expressing from within your pain (how can you not, right?) without putting thought into it.

Have no preconceived notion of what the painting is going to look like or even what the specific content is.

It may express your whole pain story, or how you feel about it, or some aspect of it. An image may appear magically within what seemed to be random lines and shapes. Or the colors and lines may remain totally abstract with nothing recognizable in them.

Accept whatever comes up as an expression of the inner life of your pain, even if it's dark and messy. Especially if it's dark and messy.

Here are some cues you can use to begin:

- Imagine you give pain the brush. What kind of art does pain make?
- Step into the feelings and emotions you have about being in pain and let them direct your brush.
- Paint how you see your pain.
- Paint how you think your pain sees you.
- Paint the story your pain wants to tell.
- Paint the truth about your pain (its depth, its meaning, your hatred of it) that you think you could never tell anyone.

EXERCISE REVIEW: IMAGING PAIN'S FORM

1. Calm your mind and body.
2. Tune in to your history with this pain.
3. Express from within your pain.

26   Giving Pain What It Wants

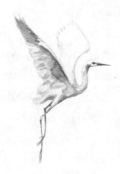

This exercise comes from my total frustration at being in pain for such a long time. I wanted to understand, once pain had sent its original message to let me know that my body was in trouble, what other purpose it could possibly be serving. What, after all this time, did pain *want* from me?

Asking this question led to looking at pain as a messenger not only of the body but of the inner self as well. If pain had already served its original purpose, I wondered if its longevity could be serving a further purpose, one that was of a more emotional, mental, or even spiritual nature. What was the deeper meaning of continued pain, and how did it relate to my life story?

🕊 EXERCISE: GIVING PAIN WHAT IT WANTS

1. Imagine Pain as Part of Your Life Story

Imagine, just for now, that your pain represents part of you that has been waiting to be heard, seen, paid attention to, respected, honored, or acknowledged.

This part of you or your life story didn't necessarily create the pain you're in, but it is possible that the pain you're experiencing right now might be helping to *express* some other long-buried emotional, psychological, or spiritual pain from the past that has no other outlet, as if some part of you is using the pain as the only channel available through which to have a voice.

2. Imagine What Pain Really Desires

Breathe softly into the painful area and try to relax as much as you can.

Gently ask the pain what it really wants and desires.

Let thoughts and images arise easily in your mind. Just be playful with it.

Maybe pain wants freedom, or to sing in the opera, or to ride a horse on the beach. Maybe it wants to burn to a crisp and whisk away in the breeze, or sob loudly, or sink deep down into the earth until it disappears completely.

3. Give Pain What It Wants

Imagine pain getting what it wants, however that comes to you to do that.

Let it float away, or get very large and angry looking, or shout through a megaphone. Put a representation of pain in a Wagnerian opera or riding that horse or flying free or exploding or imploding.

Imagine giving pain whatever experience came to you when you asked pain what it wants, and be sure that you are giving pain what *it* asks for, rather than what you want to happen *to* pain.

EXERCISE REVIEW:
GIVING PAIN WHAT IT WANTS

1. Imagine pain as part of your life story.
2. Imagine what pain really desires.
3. Give pain what it wants.

27 Writing Pain a Letter of Complaint

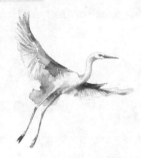

The next four exercises include creative ways I used to establish a two-way dialogue with pain.

They allowed me the sense that I was both listening to pain and, at least in my imagination, being listened to by pain. They helped reframe my experience of pain from something invasive and intractable to a sensation response that I could communicate with.

It was a way to speak directly to and with the aspect of myself that was creating and maintaining the pain in my body. It gave me useful outlets and released pent-up frustration and feelings of powerlessness.

For this next exercise, you will write a letter to pain.

If writing is not an option, you can speak your letter out loud, or into a recorder, or you can write the letter in your mind. You might also have a friend write it down for you. I prefer writing by hand because it feels more real and immediate to me, but you can do this on a computer if you wish.

Part of the purpose of this letter is to establish a relationship with pain that acknowledges a willingness to communicate openly.

Another is to clear the air, so to speak. This first communication is a chance for you to say whatever needs to be said about how pain has affected your life. This is helpful as you begin to find a way to relate to pain as a positive force.

Before you can make friends with pain, it's good to get your anger, resentment, and blame off your chest and out in the open. I've included examples of my own letters to pain throughout this book.

EXERCISE: WRITING PAIN A LETTER OF COMPLAINT

1. Begin Your Letter with "Dear Pain"

Begin your letter with the words "Dear Pain." This establishes in your consciousness that you are communicating directly with pain (as opposed to writing a journal entry, for example).

2. Don't Hold Back

Basically, you are registering a complaint with pain about your present situation. For now, keep your complaints in the present tense and only discuss what you are currently experiencing.

This can be a short missive or a long diatribe. Some suggestions:

- Tell pain how you feel about your present situation and the part it plays in that.
- Tell pain how awful it is to have it in your life. Tell it how punishing or restricting it feels, how unfair it is.
- Describe where you feel pain in your body, what it feels like in detail, and how much it hurts.
- Tell pain the things you can't tell anyone else because they will be scared for you, or feel pity for you, or try to fix it for you, or not believe you, or not understand in some way.

3. Read Your Letter Aloud to Pain

Write until you feel done. Once you are complete, read your letter aloud to pain. Imagine that pain is your audience and direct your voice toward it in whatever way that makes sense to you.

4. Assume You Have Been Heard

Assume, even though pain has no known address, that your message has been received.

After all, pain is totally accessible to you at the moment, so it really isn't far away. It's very much within listening distance.

You can send a letter of complaint to pain anytime you feel the need.

EXERCISE REVIEW:
WRITING PAIN A LETTER OF COMPLAINT

1. Begin your letter with "Dear Pain."
2. Don't hold back.
3. Read your letter aloud to pain.
4. Assume you have been heard.

28 Pain as Messenger

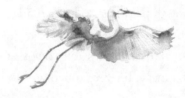

This exercise allows you to interact with pain as a messenger, and a bearer of gifts, however difficult these gifts may be to receive graciously. Pain is certainly a messenger of the body, and we understand its signals when it is telling us about some immediate physical danger or malady. I believe that continued pain can also be a messenger from other levels of the self.

In my experience, it's as if the physical pain signals, since they are insistent and unmistakable, sometimes act as a kind of carrier for other signals from deep within the self. These signals come from buried emotions that may be so numbed, covered over, or distant in time that they seem to no longer have a presence in our lives, yet if they remain unresolved, they live on in the subterranean aspects of the self.

These deeper messages have been trying to get out, or be delivered, sometimes over a long period of time. If they're still there, it may be because we have ignored them, or not understood how to hear them, or mislabeled them.

It's as if some of our older pains — our long-buried sadness, fear, anger, or loss — may be taking this opportunity to speak up through the physical pain in the body. For me, this doesn't mean that the old emotional pains are necessarily creating the physical pain, as some believe, but that they are, in a sense, catching a ride with it into our attention.

This only makes sense if we remember that we are fully integrated systems. Our bodies, emotions, and thoughts share the same living quarters. They are completely interdependent systems. These old emotional hurts want to be resolved and released, and they may take the first opportunity that presents itself to have a voice.

If we insist that our pain is purely physical without exploring further, I believe that we are not only missing an opportunity for healing on deeper levels, but we may be contributing to keeping the pain in place, as I discuss in part 2, "The Emotional Life of Chronic Pain."

One gift in the pain message, then, can be this further release, this freeing of old news.

🕊 EXERCISE: PAIN AS MESSENGER

1. Imagine Pain at Your Door

Imagine you hear a knock at your door and you go to answer it. Pain is there to greet you.

It is your specific kind of pain as a personal messenger. Take a good look.

Is pain an individual, a demon, an animal, or some other form? Does it shift around, unwilling to take a single shape?

Notice how tall it is, how much space it takes up, how light or dark, whether it looks male or female, and whether or not it seems familiar through mythology or in some other way.

2. Greet Pain

Greet pain politely. Does it step in the door or stay outside? If it stays outside, invite it in, however briefly.

Does it have a verbal or written message? Perhaps it is entirely symbolic. Does it bring a gift or someone else along with it?

3. Take What Pain Brings

Allow pain to deliver its message or gift, whether verbal, emotional, telepathic, by impression, or by offering you something or someone.

Take whatever pain offers graciously, thanking it, and letting it know you will honor it and its gift by paying some attention to what it has brought you today.

Spend as long as is comfortable for you to be with whatever pain brings you.

Look at it, feel into it, recognize it, hate it, love it, but do not try to change it just now, and try not to reject it. Let it just be what it is.

Some kind of understanding is here for you. If that is not clear now, just be with that unknowing for the moment and trust that it will reveal itself later.

EXERCISE REVIEW: PAIN AS MESSENGER

1. Imagine pain at your door.
2. Greet pain.
3. Take what pain brings.

29   Telling Pain Your Story

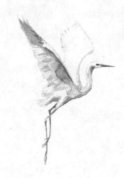

In this exercise, you will imagine pain as an entity present in the room with you, and you will use this opportunity to tell it the story of your suffering. Address pain as if it were a conscious entity.

This communication is different from writing the letter because you are no longer venting your displeasure at pain.

The purpose here is to tell your story to pain more neutrally, without animosity or blame, as if pain were a caring presence.

EXERCISE: TELLING PAIN YOUR STORY

1. Imagine Pain as a Being

Conjure up an image of pain in any way that works for you (as a shape, a color, a form, a person, a mythological god or beast, the one that came to the door in the last meditation, or a different form). Create a representation of pain by either drawing a picture of what pain looks like to you, using a small stone or other object, or simply writing the word *Pain* on a card or paper.

2. Tell Pain Your Story

Place the representation of pain across from or next to you, or simply imagine that pain sits in an empty chair across from you.

Begin to communicate, either out loud or by talking to pain in your mind. Tell your story as calmly and clearly as you can. If you are mobile, you can even act out or dance your communication. Tell pain the story of your intimacy with it dispassionately, as you would relate a news report.

3. Imagine You Are Heard

Imagine that pain hears you. Don't expect a response right now. Just let pain take it all in, so to speak.

EXERCISE REVIEW: TELLING PAIN YOUR STORY

1.   Imagine pain as a being.
2.   Tell pain your story.
3.   Imagine you are heard.

30 Listening to Pain

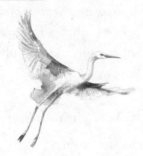

Now that you have expressed yourself to pain in a number of ways, it is time to give pain the space to speak for itself.

This exercise can be revealing of how you hold pain in your body and life, what meaning it has for you, and the possible correlations it has with other aspects of your life.

When pain is holding attitudes, emotions, and stories for you, it cannot easily leave. Once you find out what these are, you can take them back and address them directly, deciding how you will complete, revise, or release them.

This exercise helps you to more fully respect and honor pain as having a positive purpose in your life. Once pain is respected and honored, it may not have to shout so loudly for attention.

✒ EXERCISE: LISTENING TO PAIN

1. Invite Pain for a Chat

Place your representation of pain (see the previous exercise, "Telling Pain Your Story") across from or next to you. If you are mobile, you can get up and go sit in pain's place and speak for it.

2. Allow Pain to Tell Its Story

Address pain respectfully, and ask it to speak for itself. Just pretend, let it flow, and see what comes out. Here are some ideas:

- Ask pain what it is doing in your life right now.
- Ask pain what it wants from you, what it expects of you.
- Ask pain what it is better than. (What are the alternatives to being in this level of pain that are worse than having the pain?)
- Ask pain what it requires from you to heal.
- Ask pain what its positive purpose is beyond just signaling that something ails you physically. What is pain trying to give you?
- Ask pain how it wants to be respected, heard, represented, or honored.

Allow yourself to answer as pain. Just imagine yourself as your pain and go with what comes through. Make notes right afterward to review and consider later.

You can do this process at different intervals along your healing path. You might want to take each of the questions above and do them at a different time.

EXERCISE REVIEW: LISTENING TO PAIN

1. Invite pain for a chat.
2. Allow pain to tell its story.

PART 4

When Pain
Is the Teacher

31   Resistance Is Futile

One sure thing about pain is that it automatically causes you to resist it. It is something you push against, that you don't want, that you want to end.

This is a natural reaction, of course. Pain is unpleasant, even unbearable at times. It can feel all-encompassing, as if it were swallowing your well-being inside itself. I understand that completely.

On the other hand, what happens when you push against something? The wise adage "what you resist, persists" seems to be true.

The act of pushing against pain, against any situation, against another person's behaviors, anything, actually serves to hold the thing you're resisting in place.

It's almost as if, because you are putting pressure on something energetically, it must fight back to maintain its existence, and thereby the two pressures lock together in a stalemate.

Still, you may be asking honestly, *Why wouldn't I resist pain?* To not resist seems illogical. *I don't like feeling it; it's awful. I don't want it in my life, so I'm certainly not going to wel-come it. If I don't resist it, if I don't try to end it, it will take over. It will stay and stay.*

This doesn't seem to be the case, however. Not in terms of pain, and not in terms of other situations we resist in life.

You don't like pain. Believe me, I know. You don't have to like it. But it's here. The situation is here. The illness, the injury, has already happened. This isn't where you want to be. Pain isn't what you want to feel. Understood.

But pushing against it doesn't always work. Saying you don't want it over and over, trying to fight against your body or the pain or the situation, does not help. It actually hin-ders the healing process.

Pushing against pain includes labeling it as inherently bad, evil, unworkable, a punishment, a terrible burden you have to carry, or your penance for not being perfect.

You get the picture. Anything that feels like martyrdom, self-pity, recrimination, blame, accusation, or criticism is pushing-against, is resistance.

Our culture tends to adopt very polarized thinking. If it's not *this* way (on one extreme end of the spectrum), then it's *that* way (at the opposite end of the spectrum). So it might feel that if you don't resist pain, then you have to enjoy it.

But that's not so. The antidote to resisting pain isn't running around trying to welcome more pain into your life. With just about anything, there is a middle road between the two poles.

Resisting pain looks like this:

I don't like this.
I'm in a battle with you, Pain.
Go away.
I will kill you with pills.
I will avoid feeling anything at all so I don't have to feel you.
I will fight you to the death.
I hate you, you've ruined my life.

The middle road looks more like this:

This doesn't feel good at all. In fact, I feel pretty terrible, but I accept the situation for what it is, and I'm working with my pain to see what I can do to heal more quickly, to understand why it's here.

You are not denying that you are in pain, and you are not pretending everything is a bed of roses, either. You are in the middle ground that looks at everything with a clear eye, takes stock, makes some sensible and reasonable choices for that day, and doesn't insist that you've failed if you haven't healed by a certain time frame.

The path is the path. It takes the time it takes. Hating it, thrashing around inside your head about what a stupid mistake this all is, or asking over and over *Why me?* is generally fruitless.

Spend a few days doing that if you wish, just to get it

out in the open. Gently notice how much closer you are to healing. Then just let it go. Let it go.

When you are resisting, pushing against, trying to get rid of pain, it is as if you are resisting, pushing against, or trying to get rid of a part of yourself that you don't like. It's not going to work.

Pain is present in your body for a reason. Instead of trying to get rid of something that is currently an unpleasant part of your experience, it works better to acknowledge the fact that pain is part of your reality at the moment, and then to work to transform and transmute the experience.

This doesn't mean that you shouldn't take pain-relief medication if that works for you, of course. But it has everything to do with *how* you are dealing with the pain and *how* you are using medication.

Medication can be used to resist pain, to destroy it, and sometimes as a way not to have to feel anything at all. Pain relievers can also be used judiciously to help the nerves calm down and the body to get some rest so you can focus on healing.

In our goals-oriented, task-oriented culture, we often feel we have to make things happen. But pain doesn't seem to respond well to muscling our way toward healing. It just doesn't. It seems to require more softness toward the self.

32   Having Compassion
        for Yourself

When we speak of compassion, we most often refer to it as a feeling we reserve for others: others who are less fortunate, others who have lost someone or something dear to them.

We are rarely encouraged by our religions or philosophies to have tenderness and loving-kindness toward ourselves. Yet it is vital to become our own best friends when we are living in pain.

The first thing to accept about what you are undergoing is that your emotional reactions to your situation are not wrong or unnecessary.

Absolutely nothing is wrong with you for feeling the way you feel. You are not overreacting or oversensitive if you find yourself often in tears or filled with rage and frustration at what happened or is happening to you. You are not weak or silly or self-pitying.

It is normal and natural to feel strongly. Something big has happened in your life to cause the degree and tenacity of the pain you are in. It might have been sudden, or it might have developed slowly over time. Either way, the change in your life is real, the pain is real, and your feelings are real.

Having compassion for yourself means allowing yourself to feel the deep emotions that arise from living in pain and, once you have acknowledged and felt them fully, to let them go.

Besides allowing your strong feelings about your difficult situation, please understand that you are not wrong for *being* in pain. This is so important to understand and to *agree with* within yourself. It is very hard to heal when you are fighting with yourself.

Likewise, remaining in pain for some time does not mean that you are a failure. You are always doing your best. Sometimes that looks like getting up and taking a walk, and sometimes it looks like staying in bed.

Often we find ourselves the hardest to truly love, yet one of the things that pain demands from us, if we are to move beyond it, is to find a way to care for ourselves by holding ourselves gently and seeing ourselves with kinder eyes.

33   What I Learned from Pain

It took years for me to give up trying to deny or erase my experience of pain instead of letting myself truly feel what my body was carrying, communicating, and wanting to release.

Pain seems to be full of paradoxes, and one of them is that the more you try to get rid of it, the more it refuses to budge. It's like trying to cut something out of reality that's right in front of you.

It takes a huge amount of energy to not look, to keep avoiding, or to walk around it instead of just looking right at it and talking with it.

By facing pain, listening to it, and allowing it the room it was demanding anyway, my body began to relax a bit around the pain. I stopped clenching quite so much, I stopped saying no, no, no, and I began to accept.

Pain seems to require a certain level of honest respect, a bow to its mission, before it will move on. I had to let myself fully *arrive* in the situation, my condition, and the pain before I could expect things to begin to shift.

Therefore, it seems that we may not be able to get out of it until we've allowed ourselves to be fully in it.

I learned to, in a way, turn toward the pain rather than push off from it. I found ways to *include* it in my experience, no matter how much I disliked it, rather than expending energy uselessly trying to *exclude* it.

I learned that constantly saying no to pain locks things in place. Relaxing into acceptance allows the possibility for the body to regenerate.

It's like when you're a kid learning to swim, and for the first time you understand how to trust the water. You have to fully let go in order to experience the fact that relaxing will not drown you, that trusting the water is the way you enlist it as an ally.

I had to learn to stop being so hard on myself. I let go of needing to be the perfect patient. I stopped trying to live up to anyone's timetable for healing and recovery of health, including my own.

I started living more in alignment with what was true for me that day, even if it meant doing very, very little. Instead of pushing toward wellness, I learned to relax more and accept the fact that healing was going to take much more time than I would have ever imagined at the onset of this journey.

After having been in pain for so many years, I am convinced that pain brings many unforeseen and unacknowledged gifts with it.

Most of these gifts were unwelcome at the time, but looking back, I can see what I've learned from the experience of living with pain.

I found that there really was no positive way to live with pain without drastically changing my lifestyle, my attitudes, and my perceptions. These lifestyle changes and realizations were forced on me by pain; I never would have chosen this path, and pain is a very unforgiving mentor. I am, nevertheless, grateful for everything I learned.

I would have wished to have gotten to these understandings differently, but this was simply not the way it happened. Perhaps life was trying to give me these realizations in other ways for a long time before I was injured, and I was too stubborn to make the changes necessary in order to receive them.

I might not have changed in these ways otherwise, but now that I've had to in order to cope with pain, I realize they are all valuable lessons and approaches to life that are positive and healing on multiple levels.

Slowing Way Down

One of the gifts pain brought me was that I had to slow way, way down and move only at the speed that worked for my body, not at the speed that worked for my former lifestyle. I had to become what I think of as very Zen.

Pain forced me to operate in a completely different rhythm than I was used to. Life became simple, minimalist, quiet, and slow. This was a pace I normally found boring and unproductive, but slowing down taught me how to tune in to my body and its natural rhythms.

It also taught me to appreciate what is right in front of me, to enjoy what is available to me, instead of chasing after something else (mostly because I couldn't).

I found that life is richer when you slow down and take each thing as it comes. I discovered that I already had most of what I thought I should be running around getting more of anyway.

Honoring the Present Path

Another gift from pain was learning to live much more in the present. Whether we like what is happening in the present moment or not, pain forces us to be there while we are feeling it. In that way, it is a very difficult teacher.

We are brought right slam-bang into the center of *now* when pain is screaming its loudest. There is no outlet, no place to run and hide where you can't feel it. It is like spiritual training on speed.

Pain teaches us to remember our bodies, to tune in to time (because it moves so slowly), and to be *aware* right here and now. This is beneficial because we tune in to the life we're living.

We're not actually ever going to be living in the future. We're always only ever going to be living right now, so tuning in, getting present, and paying attention actually creates a richness to our life experience that is unprecedented.

At first, with pain as the mentor, it's not all that agreeable to be in tune with the present, but we learn to find the pleasant and happy things that are available right now even when pain is there, too.

We can learn to focus on the things we want to experience more of, rather than on the negatives.

In this way, despite our vehement protests to the contrary, we find out that pain *is* the path. What is happening right now in the pain *is* our healing path.

As simple and as difficult as that.

Letting Go

Pain also taught me how to let go. It forced me to finally give up the fight. It simply refused to budge until I had made an inner movement in attitude from someone who insists on making things happen to someone who gives up the need to control everything.

In this book, I discuss finding and making certain decisions in order to release feelings of victimization and powerlessness. This is so important for those of us who have felt as if outside systems hold more authority and influence over our lives than we do.

At the same time, as we take up responsibility for ourselves, we need to let go of the fight for absolute and complete control over how our bodies will heal and in what time frame. It's a balance.

We want to recognize the places that we do have a say about on a daily basis: which doctors we see, what kinds of healing modalities we choose to work with, how we are going to organize our personal care, how we handle our relationships, the choices we make about work and family demands, and the ways we find to take care of ourselves emotionally.

We also need to recognize that we are working in tandem with a partner that we're just getting to know. Pain has its own healing agenda that we can fight against or learn to honor and work within.

I learned the hard way that healing comes faster when I let go of trying to run every aspect of how my journey through pain is going to unfold. I had to learn to share the driver's seat, in that regard.

Saying No

I also learned how to say no. I had to say no to friends often and to the things I would have liked to participate in but couldn't.

I learned to say no to requests for my time and energy that didn't truly honor my limitations, that would have left me feeling worse, even if the person asking was disappointed in me. I had to learn to put my body's needs before someone else's need to have me be there for them. Sometimes this was difficult, but it taught me a lot about how to create healthy boundaries for myself.

Speaking Up for Myself

I had to learn to speak up for myself differently. I learned to ask for help. This is not something most of us want to have to learn.

We want to be fully independent and sovereign in our lives. These are attributes we prize, particularly in this culture. Yet, when we're ailing, we have to learn that we can't do it all on our own.

And the truth is, we're never doing it all on our own. Everyone is always relying on everyone else. We just tend to forget that.

Money is our go-between, but the reality is that another person is giving us a job, another person is behind the counter at the bank, another person is packing and shipping our food, another person is teaching our children, and another person is making sure the streets are safe at night.

When I learned to ask openly for help from others, I also learned to acknowledge the existence of all the other people who were already affecting my life and contributing to it, even if I didn't know them.

I also came to understand that each of us has a voice, and sometimes it takes feeling like we don't have one, and struggling with that for a while, in order to find the courage and inner strength to finally find it and speak up. Speaking up for oneself, whether to ask for help or to communicate in other ways, is the first step in rediscovering a voice in the greater world. It's the first step to self-empowerment and, ultimately, to full healing.

Being Softer with Myself and Others

When you're fine and things are moving along in a fairly normal fashion, it's sometimes hard to have patience with either yourself or others. We expect so much of ourselves all the time, and we also place these impossible standards on others, including our mates, siblings, and children.

Being in pain, I had to learn to take care of myself differently, to have greater gentleness toward myself and what I was going through. I also began to understand what others go through when they are dealing with illness, injury, loss, or other hardships.

Everyone, including me, is always and only doing the very best we all can with what's in front of us and what's inside of us. We can never know what someone else is carrying, either in terms of physical pain or in terms of emotional stress.

Having to live with less of everything — less strength, less energy, less brainpower — taught me to be kinder to myself and kinder to others. Living with pain taught me how to give myself and others more of a break.

Appreciating the Little Things

I remember sitting in my house, my body burning and aching, and noticing a ball of dust in the corner of the room. I realized that, in the past, I would have gotten up and cleaned it. Right then, that action was more than my body could handle.

I glanced around the room and saw all the things I wasn't cleaning or couldn't keep up with. It was more than a little distressing to not be able to do the simplest things, and I realized how much we take the smallest activities for granted. We assume we will always be able to do what we're doing now physically, and we never dream that we might become hugely compromised for a while or for a very long time.

I began to appreciate how much I had taken for granted in the past. Brushing my teeth, picking up a plate of food, or driving more than ten minutes used to seem like nothing, but these were now painful and laborious.

I realized how amazing life really is and how much I looked forward to regaining any capacity for doing these things with less pain and more mobility. I remembered how I may have complained in the past about having to do something minor that now seemed like a privilege to do. It was very humbling.

Being in pain, while I would prefer not to have had to go through it, nevertheless taught me a great deal about slowing down, being more present with life as it is right now, letting go of trying to completely control how my healing would unfold, how to say no when I really needed to, how to find my voice to speak up for myself and ask for help when appropriate, how to be softer and more forgiving toward myself and others, and how to be appreciative of the smallest things in life, which sometimes are the most precious.

34   The Nature of True Healing

One of the questions that has come up for me over my long sojourn with pain concerns the nature of true healing.

We think we know what healing is, and maybe we do in a rudimentary kind of way. Healing is when the pain stops. Or healing is when the illness is better.

But when is that, really? If your pain left you tomorrow, would you be healed? Or would you just be pain-free? Is there a difference? When is better *all* better? When the doctor says so, or is there some other criterion?

I think that often we define healing as an end result only. Yet it's really hard to point to.

When am I healed? Is there a moment in which I am not healthy and suddenly I am? Or is healing inseparable from living?

It seems to me that healing is the process by which we create a new relationship with our bodies, our emotions, our minds, and our spirits as demanded by some crisis in life, whether it be illness, trauma, or injury.

Something has happened that compromises our ability

to function well and with that comes pain. We are in pain until we find a way to meet it where and how it needs to be met.

This involves change. Healing is the process of change that we undergo day by day in our efforts to reconnect with wholeness and health. It may mean letting some things go — habits, hates, hurts — and it may mean adopting an entirely different lifestyle.

One thing that seems certain to me is that healing does not happen in a particular place at a specific time.

Healing happens every moment we are aware that we need to change in order to re-create the inner balance that constitutes health.

Healing is the process of working with, dealing with, loving, and having compassion for the renewed body and the new self that is trying to emerge through our pain and illness. The process and unfolding of all of that *is* the healing.

What we can point to as our healing is right here today. It is what we choose, what we do, what we think, and what we feel right now.

There may be a first day of healing — when we choose to hold our pain, our bodies, and ourselves differently, the day we decide that we will be compassionate and attentive to what we and our bodies are trying to express and become — but there doesn't seem to be a final day of healing. In a way, it is a lifelong process.

Healing is simply the action word for health. If we are to be in health, we are always making healing choices.

What we do today creates the outcome we experience tomorrow and next week and next year. Health is the outcome we desire, and every day is an outcome of some kind.

True healing goes beyond repairing the physical mechanism. It involves all layers of the self, since as I have mentioned, we are all like a wonderfully intricate pattern of interwoven parts — mind, body, spirit, emotions — all merging and converging. The body acts as the obvious vehicle for the self, but there really is no point of separation. We are it and it is us.

Healing severe or chronic pain, I believe, includes transforming our relationship to the pain, and ultimately, it is about transforming our relationship to who we are and to life.

Healing *requires* change. The stronger the pain, the longer it has been around, the deeper the transformation that is being called for.

⁂

Dear Pain,

I have been intrepid. I have been good-natured. I have been the perfect hostess. I have slogged through day after day with you blaring in my ears, trying to hear my son past your incessant blasting, trying to breathe and relax. Trying to ignore you to get some respite, but to no avail.

Trying to hear others' true voices and respond to their true tonalities, trying not to let your awful dissonance infect everything everyone says to me. I have borne up. I have been stoic.

At first, I thought I understood why you were here and that you would be leaving soon. You were just a physical signal. Now I see that since there really is nothing to alleviate the relentless atonality of your undeniable presence, I must accept that on some level you are necessary.

Why you are necessary I can't see yet, but certainly you are an unavoidable part of my life right now, and in ways I am still unsure of, I think you must be an unavoidable aspect of my healing.

35   Enlisting Pain as an Ally

When we think of pain only as a nuisance, or even a foe to be overcome, we are in danger of losing our connection with the fact that pain is part of a natural process. It is an intrinsic part of our healing.

This is antithetical to our culture's view of pain, but nonetheless, we cannot overlook the fact that pain plays an important role. Otherwise, *it wouldn't be there.*

Well, then, what possible good does pain do? *How and why am I supposed to make friends with this demon in my body?*

Let's look at the other side of pain first.

Consider not having pain, but still having your injury, illness, syndrome, or condition. Just without pain. Think about that.

How would you know there was anything wrong? What would send you to the doctor or cause you to change the way you are with your body, your eating habits, the amount and way you exercise, the number of hours you sleep?

How would you have any indication that something needed to be addressed, *right now?*

Okay, so pain is like a traffic light in the road of life. It says, stop here and take a look at where you're headed. That much can be understood.

But why do we continue to have pain once we've stopped the car (or at least slowed down and acknowledged that we might need to take a very different route)? How could pain be a helpful ally?

First, when we mask pain with pain inhibitors, we are masking one of the few signals from our body that can actually get our attention. We have turned down the volume.

This works for us when we need to rest, of course, and perhaps even to be able to function at a minimal level.

But when we turn off the volume completely, we can't hear the body anymore. At this point, we are very capable of pushing the body past what is good for its well-being.

We will keep going, keep working, keep driving, keep on keeping on because that's what we're taught is good and right, that's what we're taught "getting better" consists of, but we will be overriding the body's normal, natural cries for help.

We will be forcing it to try to heal itself while we're living as if we're not as hurt as we are and without the necessary amount of relaxation, quiet, sleep, downtime, and not-doing that it is asking for through the pain.

When we completely override the body's pain signals, we are in danger of making its healing take longer.

When we mask the pain completely, we are creating a kind of false healing. We feel better, so we think we are getting better. But how would we know? It is my contention that using pain medications to completely eradicate pain (as opposed to taking the worst of the edge off) can sometimes cause us to go beyond what the body would put as boundaries on our physical and mental activities, deprive it of what it needs to really heal itself, and create a situation that actually extends the time it takes to heal.

It may give us an inaccurate sense of what we can tolerate because we can no longer feel the pain that tells us to stop, and we may reinjure ourselves because we simply refuse to halt our activities and be quiet.

Pain, then, can tell us when to slow down and stop. It tells us that we've gone too far for the day, that the body needs to be quiet and rest. It gives us necessary feedback on what's working and what isn't.

I had to learn this the hard way because I have a condition that worsens very quickly when I try to push against the physical limitations it imposes on me.

I had to learn that pain is an ally in that it warns me when I am making things worse. I think that is part of its job, and when we ignore it or try to erase it, we are depriving ourselves of very valuable feedback.

First, what do we all usually do when the pain stops? Simple. We go back to what we were doing before the pain began. We feel that we are healed, all is well again, and we get back in our car on the road of life and continue in the same direction. Very few of us will change our lives drastically once pain leaves. Of course not, there is no reason to.

Pain is always asking for change. Most obviously, it is

asking something to change in terms of a physical orienta-
tion toward the body, such as exercise, lifestyle, eating habits, amount of rest, or some kind of physical manipulation
that restores the body to proper balance.

But pain that is chronic, that simply will not go away, is
asking for more than that. It asks us to change our orienta-
tion not only toward our physicality but toward our inner
selves as well.

We are challenged to examine our attitudes toward life,
toward how we feel about ourselves as people, toward our
choice of work, and toward our choices around the company we keep and what we do with our time.

Chronic pain demands us to look at what we need to
let go of, or realize, or embrace in order to move into a very
different stance in life and within our inner world. In short,
pain stays because it still has something to communicate.

⚜

Dear Pain,

I think you have sapped my ability to take chances,
to believe in happy endings (and happy middles).

I have been so successful in minimizing my experience of you in order to get through the days,
in order to not be a burden on others, that I have
minimized my inner self or at least the life space that
my inner self used to occupy before you turned up.

Now I am coming out the other side needing

to find out where I hid myself, and it's not easy. I so emptied my life — so that you couldn't have it all or because you demanded all that space, I can't remember — that I now feel like I'm floating free in a void, and it's really scary.

I know I used to have an active, busy life, but that life is gone, and I can't see a bridge to a new one.

Pain, you have seemed more present, more real, more immediate than God.

36   You Are Not Your Pain

Pain is so pervasive, so enmeshed with our daily experience, that we can forget what life was like without it. We may eventually lose a sense of who we were before pain entered the picture.

When I began to return from the most intense part of my journey with pain, I realized that I was going to have to find a way to disentangle myself from it.

I couldn't find a sensation of body-without-pain, even in my imagination, and I couldn't envision a future without pain, even though I desperately desired it. I had forgotten who I was without pain, and I wasn't sure who I had become from this experience.

I certainly knew I had changed irrevocably, but I wasn't quite sure in which direction all the changes lay.

This was a scary time. Pain had become so embedded in my body, my daily routines, and my awareness that this constant companion had become too familiar, like a terrorist and his hostage.

The difficulty didn't lie in me wanting to keep pain

around like an old pal, far from it; it lay in the fact that pain had been with me so long that I wasn't sure what would be left of me when it finally departed. Would it take most of me with it? I wasn't even sure there *was* a me beyond the pain anymore.

This stage of coming out of the deepest experiences with pain is really important to recognize because there may be an unconscious push and pull on the inside. Most of the inner you is working to heal, to return to life, but some frightened part of you may be worried about the you that is going to emerge.

I found that I had to disengage my self-image and my feelings of self-worth from my experience of pain and my body's current limitations.

I had been afraid that my injury, my pain, and my being in need of assistance might be turning me into a weak and needy person. I had to realize that just because my body felt weak didn't mean *I* was weak as a person. Just because my body was in pain didn't mean I was *being* a pain. Just because my pain created new needs that I had to learn to communicate didn't mean *I* had turned into a needy person.

After a time, it may be easy to believe in pain as the only real power in life. We might shift all our choice-making onto pain's shoulders. After all, it seems to rule everything.

Many of us who have been in pain for a long time have been living in reaction to pain. We have allowed pain to become the organizing principle in life.

This seems like the only choice there is, yet a subtle but important shift seems to be necessary during the healing process: to move the responsibility, the power, and the decision making back onto our own shoulders.

While pain is certainly the reason we can't do many things at the moment, we need to be careful not to allow ourselves to think that it is the director of our lives. A crucial change happens as we begin to find a way out of living utterly beholden to pain and to put ourselves back at the center of our own lives.

As far as I can tell, the whole process of living with and releasing pain has the potential of unfolding something like this:

Pain arrives.

We resist; we do all the "right" things, including therapies and medications.

Pain doesn't leave, so we try harder to get rid of it, adding alternative therapies, prayer, more willpower, more and different medications, and so on.

Pain still doesn't leave. It may even get worse.

We try harder, repeating this cycle until:

We pay attention differently, beginning to listen to pain with respect instead of frustration. We accept that pain is staying with us for as long as it takes.

We learn to work with pain as an ally. We come to a place of honoring pain's presence and its unusual gifts.

Pain begins to relax, reduce, dissolve. Ultimately, whether it completely leaves, or it stays for some time longer, we accept all of our experience with pain as part of a greater path, and we live with more ease, grace, well-being, and inner peace.

Once I recognized that I had some fears about reentering life, working with these fears was easier. I asked myself who I wanted to become.

What new insights did I have from this journey that I could share with others? What ways could I begin to reconnect with life before I was fully recovered?

And I had to face the difficult but important possibility, how would I make sure I created a new path for myself even if I never fully recovered?

37 Some Concluding Thoughts

Always remember that being in pain is not an indicator of being less of a person than you used to be or of having lower worth as a human being in comparison to others. Being in pain is simply the path you are on.

It looks different than some other people's paths, but you are not the only one on this road. There are many, many people at this time who are sharing this road with you, for whatever reason.

Pain is real, it isn't an illusion, but it also isn't a force, a being, or a sentient entity to go into battle against and overcome.

It is important to remember to believe in *yourself* more than you believe in pain.

When you work with pain through the exercises in this book, you allow yourself to work with deeper, less-conscious aspects of the self that experience pain differently than you do on the conscious level. These aspects of self may have reasons to communicate through the pain and reasons to understand the pain experience more deeply.

Because living with pain is so demanding, and so intense, it becomes part of our identity over time. Therefore, an important component of healing, particularly if you have suffered from pain for an extended period, is to find a new sense of self in which pain is not intrinsically interwoven with your identity. Part of healing is allowing the transformation of self that is asking to happen in your life, rather than trying to find a way to return to what was true for you before the pain.

We must find out who we are now, not only in terms of the self without pain, but the self who has lived *through* the pain.

This is the person who may still be experiencing some pain but is being transformed by it and is entering a richer life beyond it. This is the person who has survived the journey, grown through the trials, and changed in relationship to self, life, and the world.

Most of the people I speak with who have had to live with hardship and pain tell me that despite the fact that they would never have consciously chosen this path, they now understand how much they have learned and grown from it in ways they never would have otherwise. They say things like: *It forced me to look where I didn't want to look. It made me slow down and pay attention to myself and to my life. It taught me what was really important to me in my life.*

Most of us are looking for the one button to push, the one pill to take, or the single change to make in our lives, and it just doesn't seem to be that simple. Living in pain is not an easy thing to do, and there is no one-size-fits-all solution, no single key, no quick fix. Living with pain over time demands that we look at our whole selves, work on creating a new relationship with the pain in our bodies, and find ways to live with it as an ally so we can move beyond it.

The person who is emerging from this pain journey has the ability to live more deeply, more wisely, more kind-heartedly, and more compassionately than many others on the planet because that person has walked in pain, through pain, and with pain and has come to know the core of themselves through this intense, unforgiving, relentlessly difficult, yet deeply transformative path. You are becoming this person.

I hope the insights, suggestions, and meditations in this book have been and will continue to be a boon to you on your journey. Remember to be kind and compassionate toward yourself and to allow yourself all the time and space you need to fully heal. I wish you all the best on your journey through and beyond pain.

Acknowledgments

My heartfelt gratitude to Dr. Tracy Newkirk for his incredible compassion, caring, and stalwart support over the years. Special thanks to Dr. Michael DeFino for his gentle and compassionate treatments the first several years, which enabled me to keep on for another day. Thank you to Dr. Carol Banquer for being such a staunch supporter from the beginning. To Rae McCauley, massage therapist extraordinaire, for the amazing gift of working on me for more than a year totally gratis. To my special friends who were there in some of the most difficult times: Rick Remsburg, Thaïs Mazur, CeCe Converse, Jane DeCuir, and Nikki Ragsdale. To my friend Marsha Madden, for her soothing touch on the massage table. To my readers who offered valuable feedback: Thaïs Mazur, Joelle St. James, Bill Shockley, Lori Shockley, and Kathleen Quinn. My heartfelt appreciation to Carl Buchheit, of NLP Marin, who taught me a tremendous amount about creating rapport with my pain and with myself as a path to release. And finally, but truly most importantly, to my son, Connor, who took over so many daily tasks from the age of eleven onward, always in good humor and without complaint, and who has been an irreplaceable and beloved support over the years, thank you.

About the Author

Sarah Anne Shockley has lived with debilitating nerve pain since the fall of 2007. Because her condition was unresponsive to existing traditional or alternative therapies, she developed a unique method of pain management and pain reduction not reliant on pharmaceuticals or medical intervention. A former university instructor, she holds an MBA in international marketing, and she is an award-winning filmmaker whose work includes the highly acclaimed documentary on disabled dance, *Dancing from the Inside Out*. She is a Master Practitioner of Transformational Neurolinguistic Programming (TNLP), a highly effective methodology for releasing long-term emotional and physical pain. She lives in the San Francisco Bay Area.

Please visit the author at
www.thepaincompanion.com.

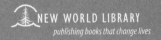